THE JOY OF SLEEPING ALONE

64 Rituals to Become the Sovereign of Your Bed & Your Life

CYNTHIA ZAK

Translated by Victoria Rojas

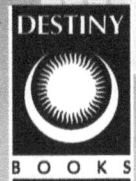

Destiny Books
Rochester, Vermont

Destiny Books
One Park Street
Rochester, Vermont 05767
www.InnerTraditions.com

Destiny Books is a division of Inner Traditions International

Copyright © 2024 by Cynthia Zak
English translation copyright © 2025 by Inner Traditions International

Originally published in Spanish in 2024 by Inner Traditions en Español under the title *El placer de dormir sola: 64 rituales para ser la soberana de tu cama y de tu vida*

All rights reserved. No part of this book may be reproduced or utilized in any form or by any means, electronic or mechanical, including photocopying, recording, or any information storage and retrieval system, without permission in writing from the publisher. No part of this book may be used or reproduced to train artificial intelligence technologies or systems.

Cataloging-in-Publication Data for this title is available from the Library of Congress.

ISBN 979-8-88850-186-3 (print)
ISBN 979-8-88850-187-0 (ebook)

Printed and bound in the United States by Lake Book Manufacturing, LLC

10 9 8 7 6 5 4 3 2 1

Text design and layout by Kira Kariakin
Illustration on pages 8–9 © Seahorse Vector/shutterstock.com
This book was typeset in Garamond Premier Pro, Agenda, Trenda, and Tomarik; ornament fonts were Moon and HWT Star Ornaments.

To send correspondence to the author of this book, mail a first-class letter to the author c/o Inner Traditions, One Park Street, Rochester, VT 05767, and we will forward the communication, or contact the author directly at **cynthiazak.org**.

Scan the QR code and save 25% at InnerTraditions.com. Browse over 2,000 titles on spirituality, the occult, ancient mysteries, new science, holistic health, and natural medicine.

CONTENTS

Acknowledgments — vii

Preface. Sleeping Alone Ignites your Intuition — 1

Introduction. The Bed All to Yourself — 3

Chapter One. The Bed of Glory — 22

Chapter Two. The Intangible Zone — 34

Chapter Three. Mantras of Empowerment — 51

Chapter Four. Divine Sensuality — 69

Chapter Five. Lucid Dreaming — 91

Chapter Six. Awaken the Heart of the World — 107

Chapter Seven. Limitless Intuitive Intimacy — 123

Chapter Eight. Welcome to Your Magic Carpet — 140

Chapter Nine. Sovereign of the Bed and Your Life — 154

References — 175

Index — 177

ACKNOWLEDGMENTS

To conceive a book, to write it, and to finally hold it
in one's hands is a miraculous process.
This achievement involves a magical interplay among countless beings
who contributed to this transformative and transcendental journey.
I am deeply grateful to the benefactors of heaven and earth.
They have cared for and guided me on this exciting
path of giving birth to a book.
The women of my lineage, the ancestral spirits of the forest, the
Sabbath-baked bread, the *mameles* and *mamushkas* beside the
samovar of tea, the invisible beings chanting mantras and praying in
Sanskrit, Tibetan, and Hebrew, angels and archangels, Buddhas and
deities whom I greet each morning—these are the powerful forces in
favor of life and joy that sustain, protect, and care for me.
My benefactors in heaven.
My benefactors on earth.
To Marlon, Allegra, and Satya, my three spectacular children,
for the unconditional love that binds and guides us.
To my beautiful friends, sisters, and brothers, companions on
journeys and in ceremonies, imbued with copal and music.
To Paulina and Ger, my literary agents at PaGe Agencia, for being there,
listening, and helping me grow as a writer and a person.
This is just the beginning, my dear ones!
To Mahar Sperling of Inner Traditions, for believing in this project
from the very beginning and for expanding its limitless possibilities.
To Beatriz, Martha, Mercedes, and the entire team of editors
and publicists who have tirelessly worked to ensure every letter
is flawless and that the book benefits everyone.
I express my gratitude to all my benefactors, both visible and invisible.
To the readers of this powerful book, which unites us inexplicably
in the mystery of dreams, the night, and its galaxies.
Thank you for being here!

Sleeping alone

is a spiritual retreat.

Repeat this mantra:
"My bed is my magic carpet.
Upon it, I perform divine alchemy
each night I sleep alone."

Your bed is your kingdom;
as its sovereign,
surrender to its mystery.

Your subtle bodies merge
into the mystery
of the night, and
when you sleep alone,
they renew your power.

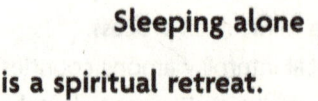

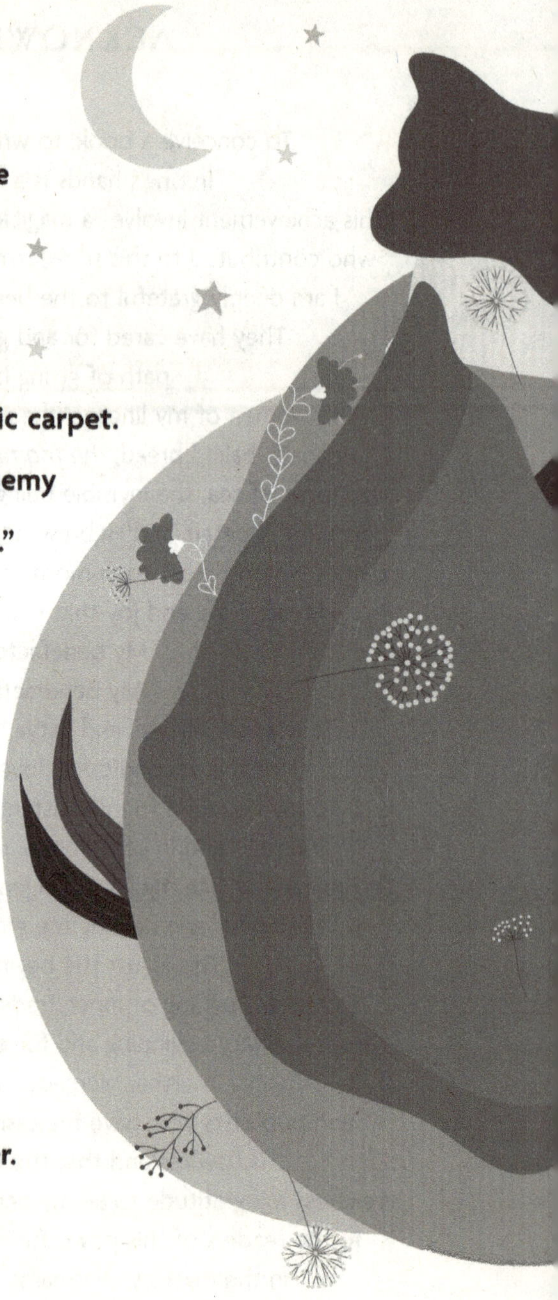

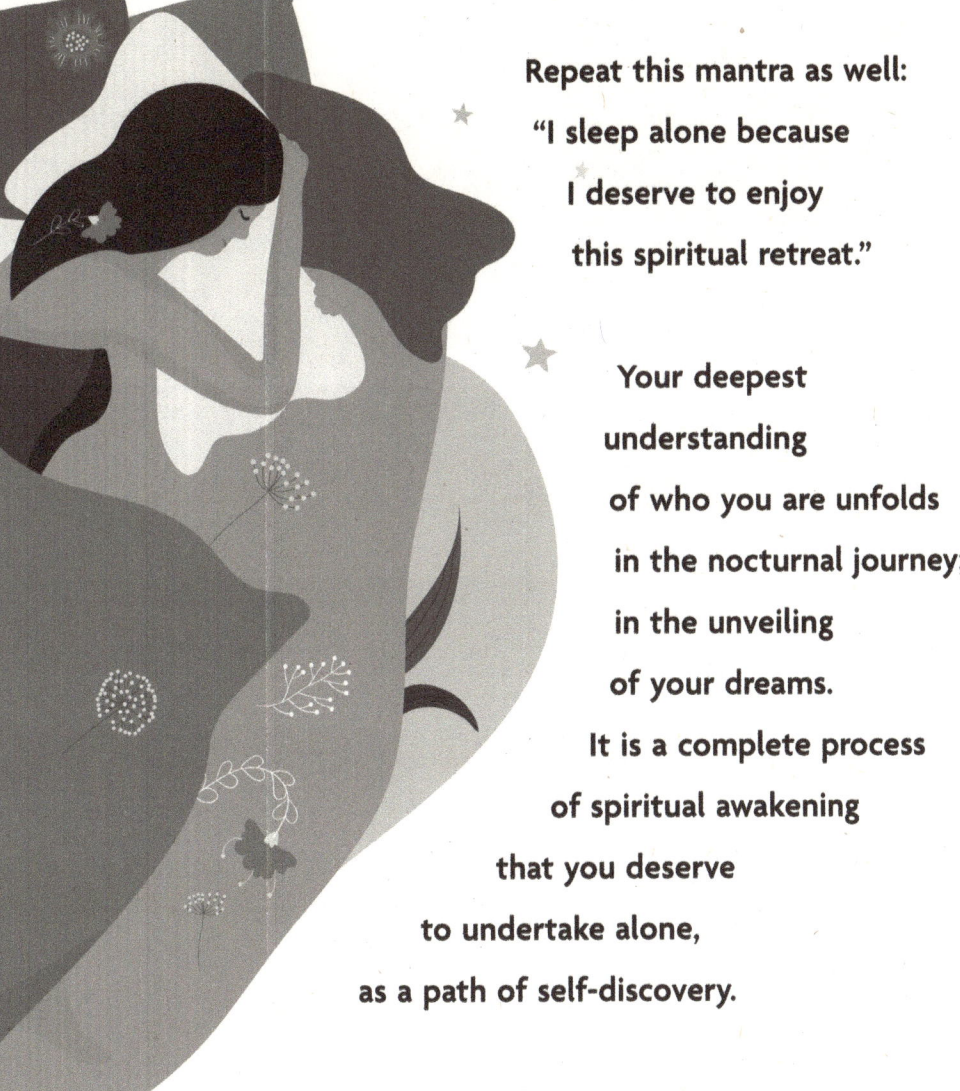

Repeat this mantra as well:
"I sleep alone because
I deserve to enjoy
this spiritual retreat."

Your deepest
understanding
of who you are unfolds
in the nocturnal journey;
in the unveiling
of your dreams.
It is a complete process
of spiritual awakening
that you deserve
to undertake alone,
as a path of self-discovery.

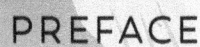

PREFACE

SLEEPING ALONE IGNITES YOUR INTUITION

Every organ, tissue, muscle, and gland in your body vibrates at a specific level. These inaudible infrasonic waves constantly emit powerful frequencies, interconnecting your breathing, heartbeat, and blood circulation. This eternal cosmogony, happening within your sacred bodily fluids and navigating your nasal cilia and veins, sustains your powerful feminine intuition.

The feminine being, endowed with an infallible and infinite capacity to see beyond, is a channel of clairvoyance that encompasses all the senses. Each organ within the body has a specific mission and function in this symphony of intuition. As the night unfolds, the orchestra of intuition within the feminine being begins to tune. During sleep, women subtly harmonize the tone, rhythm, volume, and melody of this symphony, calibrating their entire body and spirit.

For this marvel to function flawlessly, it is crucial to nurture the vessel of information—a pathway that extends from the uterus to the throat and vice versa. This process, lovingly unfolding with closed eyes as we surrender to sleep, generates new hormones and chemical balances: a gift bestowed by the majestic night.

PREFACE

In which part of your body does your ability to perceive the future reside? What sacred space of your temple resonates with the interconnectedness between your human observer and your higher consciousness?

☆ OPENING RITUAL

Before drifting off to sleep each night in solitude, embrace the opportunity to awaken new channels of awareness and attention.

1. Gently place your hands below your navel, connecting with the second chakra. This vibrant orange energy center serves as your absolute altar, deserving of reverence and honor in every moment. It is the palace of your intuition.
2. Step into your uterus—a space not of fear or pain, but of boundless expansion for your spiritual evolution. Within its depths, life, projects, ideas, recipes, songs, and poetry are gestated in direct connection with your throat and vocal cords.
3. Create your uterine altar by visualizing the sacred and magical objects that adorn it. Include anything that holds extrasensory significance, stirs your emotions, and reflects your essence as you begin to unleash your voice.
4. Breathe deeply and settle into a moment of silence. Place your left hand over your heart and gently cover it with your right hand, whispering your deepest desire to your heart. Welcome the visits of winged beings, subtle messengers who deliver precise and precious guidance and dispel any lingering doubts.
5. Empower your intuition, which unfolds boundlessly during the night and speaks from the depths of your uterus. Allow it to ignite the candles that transform you into the guide and matriarch of your own existence. Bring the wildest dreams of your ancestors to life, proclaiming your great beauty without hesitation.

INTRODUCTION

THE BED ALL TO YOURSELF

Claim your bed: expand, stretch, mark territory, explore angles and depths . . . leave not a single corner of this magical carpet uncharted.

Jump in without seeking permission from anyone.

No half measures.

No need to turn the light on or off.

Do whatever you please in your bed.

Discover and soar, without anyone attached to your experience.

Dive into your bed to create or be reborn, to dream with exorbitant clarity, to seek guidance, and to rub shoulders with the nocturnal spirits, as the queen and mistress of this sacred realm.

Surrender to the astonishment of discovering that your inner power—the balance of your physical, mental, and emotional body—needs this restorative night. When you are alone, the process of cellular repair and detoxification that comes with rest happens impeccably and without interference.

Crawl, rub, inhale and exhale; lie down in bed alone, convinced that this opportunity integrates your birth and death, your conception and your departure. All at the same time.

Delve into the depths of your mysticism—which beats in the mitochondria of your cells—and swallow your saliva to rejuvenate, taking advantage of the darkness that heals everything.

It is in bed where the pleasure of sleeping alone manifests in all its possibilities. It is here that these rituals will give you guidance and power, enabling you to discover a new connection with your being and with the universe.

By sleeping alone, you are already embarking on this path of inner growth and evolution.

Sleeping alone is a spiritual practice of high vibration, and thus it holds great power for transformation. In your waking life, you'll witness the magic that unfolds when you remain connected to your core essence, undisturbed by external energies during sleep.

IN DEFENSE OF SLEEPING ALONE

Through personally gathering feedback among women of all ages and relationship statuses (single, married, living together, separated, newly married, divorced, deeply in love, moderately in love, passionately in love, disenchanted, or fascinated with their partners), an overwhelming majority—nearly all—agreed that they sleep better alone. Many of them feel guilty about admitting this. They believe that by acknowledging this desire, they are "betraying their partners" and often they will endure more than is necessary before asking their partner to let them breathe alone for an entire night.

Some are ashamed to admit their urgent need for that solitary space.

Others are afraid of being judged and questioned by the status quo: "If you don't sleep with your partner, it's because you have problems." Women often feel obligated to explain themselves for an act of sovereignty that breaks some of the rules of Western behavior.

Many of them confess that when their partners go on trips, are away for work, take time apart, or even temporarily leave the bed, these are the happiest nights of their lives.

They crave some nights apart from their partners, a chance to breathe a few nights a month . . .

- . . . to stretch as they please,
- . . . to undress without anyone touching them,
- . . . to take up the whole bed,
- . . . to fall asleep sprawling across it,
- . . . to move as they want,
- . . . to dream without someone else's vibration intermingling with theirs,
- . . . to leave the light on to read until dawn,
- . . . to binge-watch a series,
- . . . or simply to open all the channels of the body and spirit to the pure enjoyment of sensation.

My intention with these rituals is not for you to get divorced, break up, or fight with your partner. Rather, my hope is that you will begin to discover that you can enter a sacred territory in the night journey and create an experience absolutely unique, only for you.

In fact, a 2023 study by the Better Sleep Council of the United States confirms that sleeping apart resolves sleep problems for couples.

The report found that 63 percent of couples do not sleep together for most of the night. Moreover, 26 percent of respondents said they slept better alone, and 9 percent admitted to sleeping in separate bedrooms. The same survey found that nearly two in ten Americans considered the ideal house to be one with separate master bedrooms.

HOW TO IMPLEMENT IT?

My premise, dear reader, is that you are sovereign. Start believing it and repeating this mantra whenever you remember.

Say to yourself:

- *I am sovereign and I decide when and how to sleep accompanied.*
- *I choose to listen to my hormones and the intelligence of my heart as I decide to be queen of my space.*
- *I embrace the freedom to choose solitude or companionship in my sleep.*

You can also record yourself on your phone saying: "I am not afraid to express my truth and my desire to seek undisturbed rest, without the interference of someone else's movements, smells, noises, or sounds that influence my nocturnal practice."

Having said that, establish why you want to embark on this journey and, above all, understand that what you will do is a detoxification of centuries of cultural, educational, and ancestral impositions. But, most importantly, remember that you have every right to sleep alone.

This practice is beneficial for your body, mind, and spirit at the highest levels; through this work you will start to notice and activate those benefits.

If you already sleep alone, use the rituals to understand what happens to your mind and body at a cellular level; if you sleep with someone else, you could start sleeping alone once or twice a week.

Remember that this is a spiritual practice with great benefits and that, like any inner path, it requires responsibility and determination. Of course, be very mindful of what you want and need from this work.

Separate rooms are a blessing.

Separate beds are a wise choice, but they are not ideal, as they still keep the other's energy too close each night.

The truth is that, with whichever option you choose, it is very important to explore the wonderful and unique opportunity to sleep alone in order to find yourself in other dimensions.

☆ ☆ ☆ How to Use This Book ☆ ☆ ☆

Use these rituals as you please. This book is your oracle and you can open it to any page, read it backward, follow the instructions of each of these techniques, or connect with your intuition and feel in your body and emotions which way is best for you.

Remember that this is for your enjoyment and evolution, for your connection with the great mystery and the source of wonder.

> Let yourself float, flow, and surrender to the delight of each of the nights alone that you have at your fingertips.
>
> In addition, I invite you to explore my work, which can be found on all digital and streaming platforms by searching my name. I have been playing music and instruments since childhood and over the years have compiled a vast collection of songs, melodies, meditations, and guided visualizations. Please visit my website for information about my live events and retreats, **www.cynthiazak.org**.

WHAT IF YOU DON'T HAVE THE SPACE OR THE OPTION TO SPEND A NIGHT ALONE?

If you don't have a room to sleep alone, start to see your alternatives within the situation you live in. Be creative and don't despair—simply proposing to try a night alone is already a great step on your path of evolution.

For example, consider having separate mattresses in your room so you can sleep without anyone touching you. This way, even if you share your room, you will already have more autonomy, and you will be able to start feeling the benefits of this practice in your body. If this is impossible and you must stay in a shared bed, you can engage in spiritual practices to create and activate energetic space and distance around yourself.

Sleeping alone is a spiritual and hygienic act; therefore, it is related to the cleansing of your physical body as well as the subtle bodies that surround you.

In order for you to generate this energetic distance, the first thing you will need to do before going to bed is to take a bath or shower. Wash your body consciously; you must be present in the act of removing and releasing dead cells, bacteria, remnants of the day, pollution, and toxins. As you bathe, request that you may clean every corner and, at the same time, talk to the water so that it fills you with grace and energy, creating an invisible barrier on your skin from head to toe. Do not forget to wash between your fingers, armpits, neck, and areas that you normally do not touch during the day.

Dry yourself gently with the intention of caring for your body's invisible protective layer—you are generating an absolutely unique and personal energy field that you complement when you put on your pajamas and get into bed.

Your intention is your guide—you have decided to spend the night alone even if you have someone next to you. With your skin protected, now, before sleeping, bring a request for light and glory to your whole being, activating your inner power and calling your visible and invisible benefactors. Breathe with your head on the pillow; visualize your body fully cared for and supported by forces greater than human and ask for lucid dreams that give you good news, that rebirth you with each breath. You will see how the physical presence of another being next to you will be blurred, and your experience of sleeping alone will be incomparable to anything you have experienced so far.

In this way, you are capable of creating the energy of sleeping alone even if you have to sleep with someone else. New synapses will form, strengthening your neural circuits and deepening your understanding, so that you have total success during the night.

A BRIEF HISTORY OF THE BED

Beds and mattresses are as old as humanity itself. Understanding a bit about their history and evolution gives us a means and a cosmological vision to be able to carry out our nightly spiritual retreat without qualms and without the need to ask for anyone's permission.

As everything is interconnected, the history of the bed reflects how we interact with the body at the moment of letting go of everything—when no vestiges of daytime tensions or emotional burdens remain in the muscles.

To sleep and let go . . .

That moment of surrendering consciousness—when we enter the state of sleep and shed the armor of reason—connects to the history of the bed and its role in human relationships.

Historians point to the oldest known bed, dating back a remarkable twenty-three million years to the Miocene period. This shift, where our primate ancestors moved from branches to wooden platforms, improved their sleep and potentially led to more consistent REM (rapid eye movement) cycles, impacting memory and reasoning.

Deeper dives into the unconscious and the potential for higher spiritual levels are linked to increased REM sleep. Therefore, it is essential to prioritize practices that enhance REM.

Could it be that transitioning from arboreal sleep to ground-based rest on platforms marked a turning point in evolution? This shift might have paved the way for the emergence of more advanced beings, as it fostered the development of higher awareness and the rise of spiritual seekers grappling with consciousness and existential questions.

Sleeping on the ground was transcendental for the evolution of humans—a point of no return, marking a before-and-after in the development of intelligence and consciousness.

Picture our ancient ancestors descending from the precarious slumber of the trees. No longer jolted awake, they lay upon the ground, eyes closed, finding solace in the fire's glow. This marked the beginning of a profound ritual: the astral journey, in which flesh and bone surrender their familiar form, dissolving into something vaster—incomprehensible but essential.

Etched on cave walls, their dreams took tangible form. These shared ancestors, our collective forebears, recognized a potent truth: dreams carry a pure, vital message demanding attention and interpretation.

How did sleep improve further? Seventy-seven thousand years ago, leaves, grass, and plants, known for their insect repellent qualities, were the first mattresses found in caves in Africa. From then on, the bed and the mattress evolved alongside humanity.

The Egyptians created wooden beds with legs to ward off insects and rodents. They adorned the beds of nobles with jewels and ornaments and made simple ones for the commoners. Thus, the bed became an object of social status.

Wealth dictated the level of comfort: the affluent would have wool mattresses and cloth sheets while others made do without such luxuries.

Yet, regardless of economic status, the experience of physical detachment during sleep remained uninterrupted.

The history of waterbeds stretches back over 3,600 years. Legend has it that the Persians pioneered a waterbed that used goat skins filled with sun-warmed water, possibly for therapeutic purposes.

Roman elites pioneered metal beds, feather-filled mattresses, and curtained enclosures with gleaming rails that offered both privacy and a touch of grandeur. Magnificent ornaments, soft springs, and special fabrics transformed the bed into a true ode to the ship of dreams.

This very human urge to close our eyes and drift into another world has fueled a constant evolution in sleep technology. From the elaborate beds of the Romans to today's smart mattresses, temperature-regulating sheets, and endless options for customization, long have we sought the most comfortable environment for that essential nightly journey into unconsciousness.

A bed, a spaceship: the rocket that takes us from time immemorial to the beyond.

BEDS: TOGETHER OR APART?

In ancient times, beds were communal and could measure up to six meters. In them, everyone slept together in a jumble. The whole family—servants and masters, adults and children—all in the same nocturnal space.

In inns and shelters of the past, travelers typically shared beds with roommates. The option of sleeping alone was uncommon.

As advancements unfolded, personal space gained increasing importance. Royalty, for example, began to utilize separate beds—the queen's and the king's. This marked a consistent division between rich and poor. Thus, social and economic status dictated not only comfort, but also the very act of sharing a sleep space.

However, in the mid-nineteenth century, everything changed. The ferocious spread of diseases and plagues prompted doctors to start recommending independent sleep as a means to prevent the transmission of contagious fluids. In 1880, Dr. B. W. Richardson advocated for a new approach to sleep, discouraging children and adults from sharing beds, citing concerns about adults drawing away vital warmth from children and the unpleasantness of "pestilent and heavy morning breath."

From these developments, the physical separation of bodies brought another unexpected result: women began to realize that they did not want to be passive recipients of their husbands' sexual desires. At the end of the nineteen century, the phenomenon of "the new woman" emerged.

This new woman gained a higher level of autonomy as she left the large matrimonial bed where sex was commanded by the man and embraced a new dynamic in which separate beds encouraged dialogue about the desires of both parties. The separation—that middle space between the beds—redefined their relationship, equating the partners in a new way and profoundly impacting the female psyche and women's empowerment.

The two-step space between beds was an entire universe. Crossing it or choosing to remain alone would have been an act of high symbolic power—especially for women discovering the flow of free will.

Next, the Industrial Revolution ushered in a new era of efficiency. Maximizing space and time became paramount as factories demanded a standardized and rigorous workday. To accommodate the influx of workers migrating to cities, a strategy emerged: the matrimonial bed. This approach aimed to pair individuals, often spouses, ensuring both partners adhered to the same demanding work schedules.

At this time, society has adopted a masculine circadian rhythm, or twenty-four-hour time cycle (see Stages of Sleep on page 14)—a structure based on the male physiology that once again leaves women subjected to a shared nocturnal space with limited options.

Research indicates subtle but significant differences in circadian rhythms between men and women, with women's circadian periods slightly shorter, and their melatonin and body temperature rhythms set earlier, leading to a preference for earlier sleep and wake times

Now, moral expectations, a strong sense of duty, and the fear of judgment play a very strong role in sustaining the couple. Daring to sleep apart can be misconstrued as a sign of marital discord. It is under these conditions that women submissively crawl into bed with their partners.

Women no longer have a sense of their rhythms, cycles, or hormonal temperatures because the day is marked by masculine time and the night, by obligation, has the bed as its common ground.

Curiously, Victorian-era physicians warned that sharing a bed would cause the weaker sleeper to drain the vitality of the stronger one. While an invisible exchange, it was one that they believed to leave undeniable traces on daytime mental and emotional health.

What is happening now? The National Sleep Foundation in the United States published a study relaying that 63 percent of millennial couples and 62 percent of generation Z couples sleep in separate beds, due to irreconcilable differences in bedtime routines and sleep schedules. In the case of baby boomers, 68 percent choose to sleep in separate beds, mainly due to snoring, but also due to the desire for personalized comfort—their ideal mattress, pillow, and sheets. This brief exploration of the bed's history reveals a growing embrace of solitary nights—the freedom to choose this nocturnal spiritual retreat, to enter the night as a treasure hunter on a sacred journey of self-discovery.

BE YOUR OWN RESEARCHER

Ask yourself these simple questions:

- What affects your sleep quality?
- What kind of thoughts, emotions, and external conditioning affect your sleep quality and how much you sleep?
- Does sleeping with someone next to you have any impact on your rest? Have you ever thought about or observed this?

I want you to encourage yourself and be aware of what happens in your body, mind, and emotions without judgement—as if you were a scientist developing data for research on the differences that arise when you spend the night alone versus accompanied. This path is essential for you to develop discernment and wisdom, without the ego's disruptive need to understand and explain everything.

Here is an example. This is the conclusion of research led by Dr. Colleen Carney, director of the Sleep and Depression Laboratory at Ryerson University in Toronto, Canada. She states that "Couples sleep better when they don't share a bed. There is a stigma in admitting this and people claim to sleep better together, but when we monitor their brains during research, we confirm that they do not enter deep sleep because they are constantly disturbed by noises or movements."

The Surrey Sleep Research Center in Great Britain is another leading research center that recommends sleeping apart. Dr. Robert Meadows, a sociologist at the university, agrees that "People believe they sleep better with someone, but the evidence shows the opposite." His department conducted research comparing how well those who share a bed sleep against those who sleep separately. His results suggest that when one partner moves during sleep, there's a significant increase in the likelihood that the other partner's sleep will be disturbed.

We need to dispel the prejudices and fears generated by this trend of "sleep divorce," where couples decide not to share a bed and room every night or a few times a week. Let's move beyond the outdated cultural norm that equates shared sleep with a successful relationship. This new worldview allows couples to explore nontraditional ways of living and sleeping in their relationship.

For many couples, sleeping separately helps to avoid sleep disruption. When sleeping together, snoring, different sleep schedules, and variations in body temperature can lead to frustration, insomnia, and exhaustion. In ancient Rome, the marital bed was a place for sexual encounters, but not for sleeping. This is a trend that many sleep specialists invite you to try.

In Canada, 40 percent of couples opt for separate sleep arrangements, according to Carney, reporting that their emotional and physical intimacy remains strong (Carney, 2009). In fact, prioritizing individual sleep needs can create a space for respect and understanding, fostering honor for the desires and time of each partner. This opens up a dimension for dialogue and communication and, finally, nourishes the magic of the bed so that you can turn it into your own spaceship to infinity.

STAGES OF SLEEP

It is crucial to understand the five stages that make up the sleep process, as our subtle and physical bodies connect in different ways during each stage. When we become aware of this sequence, the power of the spiritual retreat of sleeping alone becomes more palpable, present, and even urgent.

- **Stage One:** You close your eyes, and after one to ten minutes you might feel a pleasant sensation of falling or drifting, while your breathing slows.
- **Stage Two:** Sleep arrives lightly: your heart rate and body temperature drop, preparing to enter deep sleep.
- **Stages Three and Four:** You enter a deeper sleep and the so-called REM cycle begins, with slow brain waves in Delta state.
- **Stage Five:** You are fully in the REM state, with a higher heart rate and increasing brain activity. This is typically where dreams happen. The brain is activated, but muscle activity is almost completely paralyzed, which prevents you from acting out your dreams and hurting yourself—this is what is happening when you feel, for example, that you cannot scream or escape in the dream. You are breathing and your heart is beating, but you cannot move.

To understand how these five stages intertwine, we must examine both our biology and the worlds we simultaneously navigate in wakefulness and sleep.

Our mental, physical, and emotional bodies have tangible, coarser levels and subtle, intangible levels. Both levels are equally powerful and important when it comes to embarking on the adventure of sleeping alone.

Two internal biological mechanisms—the circadian rhythm and homeostasis—work together to regulate the time of falling asleep and waking up.

The circadian rhythm directs a wide range of functions—from daily fluctuations in wakefulness and body temperature to metabolism and hormone release. It makes us sleepy at night and controls how long we sleep for; it also controls our tendency to wake up in the morning without an alarm. The body's biological clock, which is based on a twenty-four-hour day, controls the circadian rhythm. The circadian rhythm is synchronized with environmental cues (light and temperature) in relation to the actual time of day, but continues even in the absence of those cues.

Sleep-wake homeostasis keeps track of the body's need for sleep. The homeostatic sleep drive reminds the body to sleep after a certain amount of time and then regulates the intensity of the sleep state. This drive intensifies each hour you are awake and causes you to sleep longer and more deeply after a period of sleep deprivation.

Exposure to light is among the factors that influence your sleep-wake cycle. Specialized cells in the retina of the eyes process light and tell the brain whether it is day or night, subsequently advancing or delaying the cycle of sleep. This is why exposure to light can make it difficult to fall asleep or to go back to sleep when you have woken up.

REM

These initials stand for *rapid eye movement* and are key to understanding the physical and spiritual processes that occur in the different stages of sleep. REM occurs within our biology, with profound implications for our deep emotional structures, which then influence what we dream, why we dream it, and, above all, how we use that information to transform limiting thoughts and a monotonous existence into something wonderful and surprising.

There are two fundamental types of sleep: sleep with rapid eye movements (REM) and non-REM sleep, which has three different stages. Each stage is associated with specific brain waves and neuronal activity. The sleep cycle goes through all the stages of REM and non-REM sleep several times during a typical night, with increasingly longer and deeper REM sleep periods occurring toward the morning.

REM sleep accounts for 25 percent of the sleep cycle and occurs for the first time between seventy and ninety minutes after falling asleep. Since sleep cycles repeat, we enter REM sleep several times during the night. Although most dreams occur during REM sleep, some may also come about during the non-REM cycle.

During the REM cycle, the eyes move rapidly from side to side behind closed eyelids and mixed-frequency brain wave activity is closer to that observed during wakefulness. Breathing becomes faster and more irregular, and heart rate and blood pressure increase to nearly waking levels. The brain and body become filled with energy: this is when we dream.

The REM cycle initiates in response to signals sent to and from different brain regions. Signals fire between different areas, including the cerebral cortex—the part of the brain responsible for learning, thinking, and memory consolidation. For this reason, REM sleep is considered to be involved in the process of memory storage and learning and also plays a role in helping to balance mood—though memory consolidation probably requires both REM and non-REM sleep.

Signals travel down the spinal cord, causing paralysis in the limbs. The muscles of the arms and legs are temporarily paralyzed, which prevents us from carrying out what we are dreaming. Abnormal disruption of this temporary paralysis can cause people to move while they dream. This can result in injuries, such as bumping into furniture while dreaming of catching a ball.

REM sleep stimulates the brain regions used for learning. Studies have shown that when people are deprived of REM sleep, they are unable to remember what they were taught before going to bed. Lack of REM sleep has also been linked to conditions such as migraines.

The reason why we dream during REM sleep is unknown. While some of the signals sent to the cerebral cortex during sleep are important for learning and memory, other signals seem to be sent at random. The cerebral cortex may try to interpret or make sense of these random signals and create a "story," resulting in dreams.

Only in REM

The REM stage begins. The brain is firing on all cylinders, almost like it's awake; the heart is racing, like you're on a brisk walk; brain waves are at full speed and muscles are paralyzed.

You can't move, as if you were under the influence of a psychotropic drug that your own body is manufacturing. In this magical and primitive state, control shifts, and the solitary confinement of your body becomes fertile ground for your mind to freely explore the dream world. With this knowledge, you have the potential to transform the chemicals and proteins in your body into something mystical—transcending the ordinary and accessing other dimensions.

You can only achieve this during your spiritual retreat of sleeping alone—ensuring that no one is able to contaminate what you are creating. You are an alchemist at this moment, capable of transforming iron into gold with a chemical formula that resides within your own organism. Your body does this on its own, without your conscious intervention, every night when you sleep. Now, in your sovereign place, you will claim this REM realm for yourself alone.

BRAIN WAVES

To complete our understanding of the REM process, it is worth mentioning that the brain waves that are emitted during the REM stages of sleep bring us closer to our higher self as they direct information from the Source. *Brain waves*, or encephalographic waves, are the repetitive (oscillatory) patterns of electrical activity that are generated in the different structures of the brain.

Brain waves are the means by which neurons communicate with each other through small, measurable electrical impulses. These waves have different types of frequencies: some are faster and others are slower. To reach slower waves, the physical body and breathing must be in perfect harmony, without interruptions or interventions. If they are separated through filters, we can observe them more clearly.

Five Types of Brain Waves Based on Their Vibration

- **Delta:** 1–4 Hz is the lowest frequency, associated with deep sleep, meditation, cortisol reduction, and access to the unconscious mind.
- **Theta:** 4–8 Hz is the frequency associated with meditation, deep relaxation, and creativity.
- **Alpha:** 8–14 Hz is the frequency at which the brain is focused and productive. These brain waves increase learning capacity and reduce stress; they help to relax and focus, maintain positive thinking, and facilitate the state of flow.
- **Beta:** 14–30 Hz is a very high frequency and maintains focused attention, analytical thinking, and problem-solving. It stimulates energy, action, and high levels of cognition.
- **Gamma:** 30–100 Hz waves produce attention to detail and help with memorization. They are related to innovative thinking and creativity.

NEIDAN: INNER ALCHEMY

Throughout history, humanity has sought potions and elixirs to achieve profound transformation, yearning for vitality and eternal youth. The ancient Chinese energy practice of *qigong* pursues a similar quest, but on an internal level. It focuses on three primary centers within the physical body, believed to be gateways to nonphysical realms. In the head is *Shen*—connected with spirituality and the fifth dimension. In the center of the chest is *Qi*—the energy center of *pneuma*, or the vital air connected with the fourth dimension. In the sacral area, is *Jing*—the physical body that unites us with the third dimension.

Now, lying down to sleep in your chosen palace, nothing and no one will be able to interfere with the nourishment of these mystical centers. Cultivate, awaken, and understand these centers as an inexhaustible source of vital and spiritual energy. Use these energy centers in your favor, since in the nocturnal rituals of your personal retreat they will explode with information.

WHEN YOU SLEEP BY YOURSELF, YOU THINK BETTER

To begin, it is essential that you understand the basic brain mechanisms of sleep. With this knowledge, the importance of sleeping alone will become concretely clear and evident, allowing you to use the space of sleep to activate your creative and manifesting machinery to its fullest potential. As you come to understand how your brain lives during rest hours, you will see, from another angle, the importance of setting aside time for your nightly spiritual retreat.

The *hypothalamus*, a structure the size of a small seed that is located deep in the brain, contains groups of nerve cells that act as control centers. These affect sleep and wakefulness. Within the hypothalamus is the suprachiasmatic nucleus (SCN)—groups of thousands of cells that receive information about light exposure directly from the eyes and control their behavioral rhythm.

The *brainstem*, at the base of the brain, communicates with the hypothalamus to control the transitions between wakefulness and sleep (the brainstem includes structures called the *pons*, the *medulla oblongata*, and the *midbrain*). The cells that promote sleep within the hypothalamus and brainstem produce a brain chemical called gamma-aminobutyric acid (GABA), which acts to reduce the activity of wakefulness centers in the hypothalamus and brainstem. The latter (especially the pons and medulla) also play a special role in the rapid eye movement (REM) stage, sending signals to relax the muscles essential for body posture and limb movements, so that we do not move during our dreams.

The *thalamus*, or the covering of the brain, acts as a transmitter of information from the senses to the cerebral cortex, processing information from short-term memory to long-term memory. During most stages of sleep, the thalamus remains silent so that we can disconnect from the outside world, but during REM sleep the thalamus is active—sending images, sounds, and other sensations to the cortex, which then fill our dreams.

The *pineal gland*, located between the two hemispheres of the brain, receives signals from the suprachiasmatic nucleus and increases the production of the hormone melatonin, which helps induce sleep once the lights are turned off. Scientists believe that the peaks and valleys of melatonin are important for synchronizing the body's circadian rhythm with the external light-dark cycle.

The *basal forebrain*, located near the front and lower part of the brain, also promotes sleep and wakefulness, while part of the *midbrain* acts as an arousal system. The release of adenosine (a chemical derived from cellular energy consumption) from cells in the basal forebrain (and likely other regions) helps to promote the sleep drive.

The *amygdala*—an almond-shaped structure involved in emotional processing—becomes increasingly active during REM sleep, while clusters of sleep-promoting neurons in many parts of the brain become more active as we get ready for bed. Nerve-signaling chemicals called neurotransmitters can "turn off" or moderate the activity of cells that signal wakefulness or relaxation.

LUCID DREAMING

In this book we will work with the practice of lucid dreaming. In lucid dreaming you know you are dreaming; you do not wake up, but you are aware that you are in the dream world, still asleep. You can intervene in what happens, and even change the course of the plot. When you conquer this territory, you have gained a lot of ground in the ascent of your physical, mental, and emotional intelligence.

If you are able to lucid dream, you are already capable of programming and managing at will regions and sections of your brain that were previously subject to chance and circumstances. The production of lucid dreams (because it is something you choose, you do it at will, deciding to do it) is associated with a high level of consciousness called *metaconsciousness*; with it, you can understand your own thought processes. Therefore, people with a high ability to monitor their own thoughts have a greater chance of experiencing lucid dreams.

Lucid dreamers exhibit a unique brain wave signature, a blend of REM sleep and waking consciousness. Additionally, specific areas of the prefrontal cortex, linked to complex cognitive functioning, become more active. At the same time, people who produce lucid dreams show a development of the anterior prefrontal cortex area, associated with high levels of self-knowledge and self-reflection that are activated in everyday life—you have more control over your dreams, thoughts, and ideas, you react less to stressors, you make decisions from very innovative perspectives, and you live in a creative exchange between the dream world and the daytime world.

Lucid dreams have been present in all parts of the world since the beginning of time. Literature and art in general pay homage to them, and the discovery of their depth for spiritual evolution is incalculable. In lucid dreams, you can understand, ask, comprehend, expand, change the course of events, be grateful for the future, and plant clear seeds of what you want and desire, because in the dream world you have absolute power over everything.

CHAPTER ONE

✶ THE BED OF GLORY

Just as each person eats from their own plate, it is required that each person sleep in their own bed.

A POPULAR SAYING FROM THE NINETEENTH CENTURY

Sleeping is a private, intimate, personal, and sacred act. The Industrial Revolution ushered in the idea of sleeping with one's partner, a practice that was reinforced by the church and moralistic thinking. Spouses were encouraged to sleep together as a means of demonstrating compatibility and harmony to both themselves and others.

From straw and dirt beds to the beds we use today, humanity has gone through many different expressions of sleeping—ranging from being fully dressed to sleeping naked, entire families sharing one bed, to travelers temporarily sharing beds in inns while journeying in the Middle Ages.

The history of sleeping and beds is intimately linked to human habits, and, more importantly, to the restorative power of deep sleep. When the cerebral cortex—responsible for memory, thinking, language, and more—disconnects from the senses, it enters a recovery phase.

If your brain uses 20 percent of the oxygen you inhale during the day to feed 86 billion neurons and 300 million cells, it is essential that at night you repair and recover from this oxidative stress process.

Do you think it's possible to do this organically and meditatively if someone next to you is snoring, moving, kicking, or touching you?

Women who sleep alone are more intelligent and more independent; they are queens of their palaces and the mistresses and ladies of their intuition—the indisputable guide in all their decisions.

Here are some rituals to glorify your bed: a bed of roses, a revered space for you alone, where you recharge, recover, and reclaim your wild nocturnal energy to illuminate the day.

Reclaim your right to sleep alone by weaving magic into your bed. Let the sheets, blankets, and mattress transcend their ordinary purpose. Breathe new life and energy into each element of your nocturnal journey. See them not just for what they are, but for the potential they hold. Imagine the possibilities for deep rest and restoration that lie hidden within each element.

What could those clean sheets be during the course of the golden night?

How will your pillow hold your head and its muses?

Does the comforter smell of any memories of past lives you don't want to fade?

Such is the magic of what surrounds you as you step into the deep, revealing sleep of your night, all by yourself.

☆ RITUAL 1. ENCOUNTER WITH YOUR GURU

1. Before sleep, sit down for a moment and place your pillow in front of you.
2. Bring to mind when this object came into your life, where it came from, whether you chose it or if it was given to you.
3. Meditate while placing your hands on it while breathing.
4. Visualize the pillow as a portal for lucid dreams and answers that you will receive in wakefulness.
5. You can also ask for answers and clarity on the path of your dreams. Remember that your pillow will support your head and brain, accompanying you in the expansion of your consciousness.

Purpose and How to Use It

Everything leaves an imprint on the place where you lay your head when sleeping.

The pillow becomes a guru to whom you surrender your devotion—a sacred place, almost like an ancient temple that you must enter barefoot, with the utmost respect.

If you could measure the frequency of energy absorbed by the pillow each night, you would be surprised at its strength and quality. These impressions, though unseen, hold a powerful influence, as each impulse, movement, or dream you produce is drawn or present in the pillow.

A simple pillow or headrest becomes your vehicle for a profound journey into the depths of the night and the mystery of your unconscious mind.

☆ RITUAL 2. CONQUERING THE BED

Perform the following ritual with total presence as you breathe. Try to have a pen and paper next to your bed to write down what you remember from your dreams when you wake up. Trust in the solidity of the vehicle and the freedom of your brain to establish lucid dreams as you sleep alone.

1. Remove any unnecessary items from the bed—any object that is between the sheets or on the blanket.
2. Move to the middle: seek to position yourself right in the center of the bed.
3. Lie down on your back, opening your arms and legs as wide as you can. Stretch out, conquering space; your body has no limits in the bed.
4. Breathe, feeling that midline that divides the two worlds: that of sleep and wakefulness; that of the conscious and unconscious; that of the dream world and the daytime senses.
5. Take ownership of the entire space and lie down as if your body were a four-pointed star with a glowing, beating center.

Visualize the poetic figure of your being as a diamond shining in this space.

6. Stretch your arms and legs and feel the axis that marks your heartbeat; feel its rhythm and the message it transmits to you.
7. Breathe abdominally, from the diaphragm, allowing your stomach to rise and fall rhythmically. Now, let sleep take you away.
8. You will enter a state of relaxation and creativity. Let the ideas come—don't interrupt them. If there are thoughts, let them pass as if they are clouds in the sky.

Purpose and How to Use It
The space of the bed is a symbolic place that reflects the relationship you have with the world, with objects, with the places you inhabit and pass through. Do you claim your space in the world, in your house, in your workplace? Do you expand and occupy what you deserve, or do you settle for a corner where you barely fit?

When you perform this ritual, you grant yourself permission to explore previously taboo, unattainable, or distant areas of your life. Stretching out in bed is a symbolic act of claiming your space in your waking life.

Conquering the bed is a practice that I invite you to do whenever you can (at least once a week in your nightly retreat of sleeping alone), to observe and record what happens in your body, psyche, and emotions when you wake up. Take possession of your rest spaces by opening the center of the bed as your absolute kingdom, transforming half of the bed into the axis of the world and re-educating your body to feel, in a new way, your place on the planet. You have permission to grow and expand; to show yourself in all your expressions.

☆ **RITUAL 3. ONEIRONAUT**

1. Create a firm intention to have lucid dreams. Express to yourself that this is what you want to do.
2. Remember your intention throughout the day (repeat to yourself during your waking hours that you will wake up in your

dreams), especially focusing on repeating the intention before going to bed.
3. Do a short meditation, setting the intention to observe your dreams and become aware that you are dreaming.
4. Have a notebook and pencil next to the bed, as this predisposes your being to remember the dream. Be aware that you have it available, at hand.
5. Set the alarm to wake you up two hours earlier than usual. Wake up and stay calm for ten minutes until you fall back asleep.
6. Remember the contents of the dreams and write them down.

Purpose and How to Use It

Like an astronaut traveling through space, the *oneironaut* navigates in dreams. This term is used in psychology to define someone who is aware that they are dreaming, in a mental state similar to wakefulness.

During a dream, when you gain awareness that you're actually dreaming, you enter a state of lucidity, or a *lucid dream*. This allows you to interact with the dream world, hold conversations with dream characters, and even influence the course of the dream.

Imagine waking up within a dream, like a movie character suddenly aware of being both spectator and actor. Perhaps you've experienced this—a thrilling awakening within the dreamscape. For those who haven't, or even for those who have, the purpose of this ritual is to cultivate familiarity with this state, allowing you to harness its potential.

By night, dreams weave a tapestry of shared humanity. This enigmatic blend of daily residue, echoes of past lives, whispers of infinity, and the language of wordless intuition holds boundless power—if we can learn to harness it.

When you sleep alone, you have an immeasurable opportunity to work with yourself on the spiritual path of lucid dreaming; a path that millennial cultures—such as Buddhists with dream yoga, or Hindus with yoga nidra—have practiced for centuries.

The most precise way to become an oneironaut with lucid dreams is to use the ritual's resources: minutes before bed, promise yourself to wake up in dreams; set your alarm to wake up two hours earlier than usual, stay awake for a few minutes, and then go back to sleep. Remember to have a pen and paper next to you.

As with any practice, patience and self-compassion are key. If you don't get immediate results, keep trying and, little by little, with perseverance and discipline, you will begin to enjoy the specific experience of waking up in the middle of a dream. You can start by doing this ritual once a week and, when you notice how it resonates in your body and mind, gradually increase the frequency of the practice. Meticulously record your dreams, for within them lie valuable insights about your desires and life's direction.

☆ RITUAL 4. CARDINAL POINTS

1. Spread out on the bed as you connect with the cardinal points of your being. As you breathe, honor who you are:
   - The soles of your feet represent the South, an anchor of stability intertwined with freedom.
   - Your crown, the highest point of your head, embodies the North, connecting with the universe and the messages from above.
   - The right side of your body represents the East, brimming with active energy. These limbs collaborate with the processes of the world and of life, mirroring the cycle of birth and rebirth like the rising sun.
   - The West is represented on your left side, where your heart beats a steady rhythm, holding your intelligent center of emotions and your capacity for transformation.
2. Embrace these parts of your being in their entirety, understanding that they are magnetic points of the Earth that interconnect you with everything.
3. Visualize your body as a high-vibration magnetic center in the middle of the mattress, so that these cardinal points call upon the vital energies of the planet.

4. You can hang a drawing of your body or a silhouette with the cardinal points from the headboard or ceiling above your bed, to remember that you are the compass of the world.

Purpose and How to Use It

As a navigation system, the compass uses the cardinal points to guide explorers who dare to venture into intangible areas that have no map. These are magnetic points that hold specific information for navigators, walkers, and pilgrims. Ancestral traditions give power to each of these points, demonstrating a worldview that unites and interconnects everything, reminding the practitioner or initiate to invoke the protections that surround them.

This ritual transforms you into your own compass. You'll greet the cardinal points, igniting visualization and creative imagination and honoring the life-giving elements—calling upon the Great Spirit of the sky, soaring on the wind, above. Below, visualize the Earth's heart, offering firm ground and fertile space for sowing. To your left, invoke the East, where fire ignites like sunrise. To the West, call upon cleansing water, guiding you toward balance.

At your core, your vital heart pulses with each beat. Feel its rhythm flow through your entire being—heels, legs, and even the back of your head. Though unseen, these activated areas integrate to become your own internal compass.

This nighttime ritual finds its echo in your waking life, as you can carry it present and active in everything you do. Visualizing these points and their powers will allow you to navigate difficulties or obstacles in a serene and graceful way, knowing you're supported by forces both seen and unseen.

☆ RITUAL 5. TRATAKA

1. Find a quiet space a few minutes before going to sleep. Ideally, your own bed and room are conducive to this spiritual practice of concentration.
2. Light a candle, positioning yourself so your eyes meet the flame's steady light. Breathe deeply and observe its unwavering

glow. You can use a wax candle or an artificial candle as a safer alternative—the focus lies not on the object itself, but on the unwavering beam that guides your gaze.

3. Try not to blink (this is a mechanism that requires your full attention). Look at the flame for a couple of minutes and then close your eyes.
4. Look at the image of the light in the middle of your eyebrows. Observe what appears in the space between your eyebrows, like the negative of a photo. Remain this way, enjoying the experience.
5. Continue to breathe consciously and keep looking at the flame. Let thoughts pass like clouds: you may feel many things—different emotions, thoughts of all kinds—but stay focused on your gaze and your breathing.
6. Take five more breaths with full and slow inhalations and exhalations. When you complete this cycle, open your eyes.
7. Write without thinking or correcting your experience, allowing the unconscious to come out and flow. Prepare your body, mind, and emotions to go to the world of dreams.

Purpose and How to Use It

This simple practice of observing the steady flame of a candle, a star, or a point of focused light where we can rest our gaze without blinking becomes a gateway to our inner world—to the unseen system that supports us, and, ultimately, to a broader understanding of our interconnectedness with everything and everyone.

Trataka is a Sanskrit word that means "to look, to observe." It is a yogic purification method and meditation practice that involves gazing at a single point for several minutes without blinking. This activates the third eye—the chakra that resides between your eyebrows and opens the mind to mystical experiences filled with messages that awaken dormant abilities such as telepathy, clairvoyance, clear intuition, and unconditional love for humanity.

Trataka calms and decongests mental noise.

It unfailingly calls for creative silence so that innovative ideas may reach your heart.

It produces an intangible exchange between the eyes and the information received by the brain, translating it into images you have never seen before.

By concentrating your gaze on one point, you balance your vagus nerve and, consequently, your entire hormonal and respiratory systems come into alignment.

Trataka has no contraindications, and you can do it alone or with the people that surround you at least once a day for a couple of minutes (you can start with a few seconds and expand the experience as you get more practice).

Your brain's functionality expands.

Your gaze becomes sharper and deeper, allowing you to see beyond and understand the subtlety of bodies.

Ask the flame, the fire, to answer you and allow you to see beyond the obvious and evident. Prepare for the journey of Trataka.

☆ RITUAL 6. SIT ON THE THRONE, QUEEN

1. Find a chair or armchair that you like, preferably one with armrests. Select something that you have at home to create your throne.
2. Place your throne near your bed for sitting before going to sleep. You should have it close, so that it becomes part of your furniture and your mind recognizes it as part of your nightly ritual.
3. Paint, decorate, and embellish it with colors, crystals, feathers, stones, sparkles, fabrics, or ribbons. There are no limitations, so unleash your imagination. Feel these adornments resonate with your heart's intelligence.
4. Craft your own throne to be a sanctuary that celebrates your inner queen. Here, judgment and self-criticism have no place.

Adorn this space with objects that spark joy—for it is your altar to meditation and a gateway to your profound self. Sit, rest, read, sing, breathe deeply. Feel your body; observe your soul. Ascend your throne—a vision of magnificence—ready to reign over your inner world.

5. The throne is your transitional territory between the dream world and wakefulness, between the unconscious and the conscious. Make it yours, own it, enjoy it.

Purpose and How to Use It

The transformation of everyday objects into sacred spaces is a powerful way to embrace your worth and your role in this space and time. As you practice living with the energy of the queen on her throne, an unconscious and very transformative change occurs in your belief systems. Thus, what seems to never move begins to flow. The symbolic act of creating and sitting upon your throne combats self-destructive thoughts and intelligently balances the harsh criticisms you may have toward yourself.

First, sit gently on your sacrum. It is your sacred area, the one that supports the organs that give life: uterus, ovaries, fallopian tubes, glands, and tissues perfectly intertwined with creative energy.

As you sit with regal posture, imagine your spine as a column of golden discs. Within them flows a wellspring of intelligence, a symphony of subtle energies, culminating at your crown, where you connect with infinity.

Claim your throne, Queen. At least once a day, grant yourself this solitary space. Honor it, for it is yours alone. While you are there, record the ebb and flow of emotions and ideas. Witness them gently dissolve, making way for wonders yet to be discovered.

When you feel ready to get into your bed, do so wearing your diamond crown on your head. With great respect and great honor for your being, which consciously rises with each breath, prepare to sleep like a queen. Sleep to recover, renew, balance, discover yourself, connect with invisible worlds, leave your body, and transmute toward advanced states of consciousness; meditate deeply and find answers to your daytime questions.

Use your throne to create that permanent connection between your body and soul, between your head and heart, between your desire and the concrete manifestation of what you ask for.

Mystics have long viewed sleep as a gateway to another realm. In Judaism, for instance, the morning prayer *Modeh Ani* (I give thanks) expresses gratitude to God for bringing us back from the other world—an acknowledgement that our souls, entrusted to God during sleep, are renewed and brought back upon waking.

I share Modeh Ani, which acknowledges the mystical nature of gratitude and the sense that the soul transcends the body, particularly during lucid dreaming. By divine grace, we awaken each morning as our spirit rejoins our physical form. The prayer beautifully captures this sentiment: "I thank you, King of the Universe, for with Your grace You have returned my soul to my body. My faith is great."

☆ RITUAL 7. SPEAK SOFTLY TO YOURSELF

1. Let your body fall onto the bed; feel your back well supported.
2. Place one hand on your abdomen, below your navel, touching the area of the feminine altar.
3. Place the other hand over your heart as you begin to take conscious breaths.
4. With each inhalation, feel the breath reach the center of your chest. Include a high vibration word of your choice (think of a word that makes you feel good and beautiful, and generates good energy for you and others when you think of and say it).
5. Keep the word in your mind and visualize a golden line between your lower abdomen and your heart, which moves like a constant upward spiral as you inhale.
6. Place the word you have chosen in your hands and pass it over your entire body, harmonizing your nervous system. Do this as if you were giving yourself a long caress.
7. Do this ritual as a nightly form of meditation. With this word, you are training your mind in a new habit.

Purpose and How to Use It

Speak softly to yourself, love yourself dearly, open your mind, and expand the art of being. Look ahead; feel within: you are the beacon, the light, and the air. While making a whispering sound, caress your body not only with your hands but also with your breath. Your vital force, prana, comes out of your mouth and nose every time you exhale. This air is of the utmost importance in the processes of spiritual growth, as this spirit navigates the subtle channels of breathing. Although it is invisible, it has great power.

This ritual primes your mind, heart, and intuition for a night of heightened awareness and introspection. Keep a pen and paper by your bedside to capture the chosen word and its personal resonance. Most importantly, record your dreams after this practice. The power of self-affirmation can be revelatory, surprising you with insights in the waking world. Meditation before sleep is a key to deep rest, offering well-documented benefits. This nightly practice can have a profound impact on your understanding of the human experience.

From the time of flickering fire in ancient caves, we've always sought light to pierce the dark unknown: a realm that mirrors our own unconscious. The night, with its hidden secrets and uncharted territories, ignites our sense of exploration and wonder. We gaze upward, drawn to the constellations, the moon's phases, and the vastness of the cosmos that envelops us. This darkness compels us to look beyond, to experience the awe-inspiring infinity of the night sky and the contemplation of the extraordinary. Let this ritual serve as a meditation, fostering a love for the night and your connection to the infinite. Develop your worldview by connecting your cells with the stars, your breath with the moon that moves the tides, and your being with the whole.

As you drift toward sleep, your final thought holds immense power for your nocturnal evolution. Let your last conscious whisper be a gentle caress, a testament of self-respect, and a love waiting to be explored.

CHAPTER TWO

THE INTANGIBLE ZONE

Sleeping alone challenges many social, political, and even economic rules. In many situations in life, women are still subordinate. Even in the most "harmonious" of marriages, when the woman says "NO," things don't flow quite so easily, as setting limits throws others off balance.

Sleeping with another person could put you in a quasi-permanent relationship of dependence while you establish a parasitic dynamic, which sucks, absorbs, and phagocytizes your vital and divine energy.

Between saying "yes" to sharing the bed or opting for "no" is a thin red line full of taboos. The traditional narrative often burdens women with the weight of explanation, even when the expressed desire is deeply personal.

You are free to sleep with someone if you want to.

You are free to sleep alone if you want to.

A beautiful journey unfolds from our sensory perceptions to an expansion of consciousness, where we can nourish ourselves with the invisible. Women, often adept at trusting the intangible, may find this access easier. We can learn to honor that space, known and felt more deeply with the body than with the mind alone.

As Carl Jung defines it, signs and symbols are different things. Signs offer a direct link to the familiar, while symbols hold an inherent ambiguity, beckoning interpretation and revealing the unknown.

These rituals invite you to embrace the boundless richness of symbolism—a language each of us interprets uniquely. Through this exploration, you'll discover the unwavering certainty that resides within you.

You don't have to ask anyone's permission.

Nor do you have to give explanations.

The time has come to embrace the invisible force that dwells within and beyond you. Awaken it, and it becomes your wellspring for renewal, rebirth, and revolution . . .

The intangible zone transcends a mere tourist destination. It's a pristine sanctuary, accessible only to you, where you hold the power to enter and depart at will. Here, your hormones, glands, and internal systems thrive in an immaculate environment, free from external energetic disturbances.

Here is a poem that I turned into a song, crafted to inspire and guide you as you discover the intangible zone within yourself:

> *There is a jungle within you*
> *With its rivers, plants, stones . . .*
> *So lush,*
> *pure richness you can connect with.*
>
> *Water flows through your veins.*
> *Air flows through your cells.*
> *Fire grows in your chest . . .*
> *And the earth beats in your bones.*
>
> *But if you want to awaken,*
> *you must go deeper within.*
> *But if you want to discover,*
> *you must go deeper within.*

To the intangible zone,
to the intangible zone...
That unexplored space,
the purest of your jungle...
Where mystery manifests itself.

And if you seek to understand...
And if you long to breathe...
When you need to pause,
the intangible zone awaits you.

Where there are no maps, let go.
If there are no paths, make them.
Though at first you may feel fear,
in the intangible zone you will understand.

Everything is simpler than you think.
Everything is sweeter than it looks.
Within you the answers await:
You are the master and you hold the power.

Cynthia Zak, "La zona intangible"
(The Intangible Zone)

☆ RITUAL 8. NOCTURNAL FENG SHUI

1. Clean and organize the space around your bed.
2. Remove anything you store underneath the bed, such as boxes, packages, and so on, and clear the area so that air can flow freely.
3. Remove any mirrors in front of the bed so that you do not reflect yourself while sleeping. This disperses energy.
4. Try to keep your bed against a wall and not directly facing the door (although you should be able to see the door).
5. Select a photo or image of something that is important to you.

This should be the last thing you see before bed and the first thing you see when you open your eyes (it could be a religious or spiritual image, a photo of a teacher, a loved one, etc.).
6. Place furniture in pairs: bedside tables, chairs, or anything else. Always have pairs near the bed to create balance.
7. Avoid electronic devices near the bed.
8. Open the windows every day and make sure that everything around the bed is kept clean and organized.

Purpose and How to Use It

Feng shui, which literally translates to "wind-water," is an ancient Chinese practice that cultivates harmony and balance in our living spaces. Rooted in the poetic concept of *chi*—the energy of the universe that binds all things—feng shui flourishes in environments free from physical, mental, and emotional clutter.

True vitality originates from within, influencing the order and flow of your energy outward. This extends to your sleep environment—the arrangement of your bed and objects can dynamically impact your nocturnal evolution. By creating a harmonious space, you allow your chi to flow freely during the night, empowering your lucid dreams and dream journeys.

Chi constantly influences our lives, emotions, and ideas. It flows both within and around us, weaving invisible threads of connection. In feng shui, there are five elemental energy bases to consider. After sharing them with you, I'd love for you to observe them within yourself:

- *Wood*: A noble element that promotes creativity, growth, stability, and permanence. If you want to include it in your home, you can represent it with plants, trees, and green objects. Where does wood reside within you? What part of your body does it represent?
- *Fire*: A very powerful element that represents passion, energy, expansion, and transformation. You can use candles, lights, or any representation of fire. You can also incorporate red objects

into the room. Where does fire reside within you? What part of your body does it represent?
- *Earth*: The element of stability and strength can be invited into your environment through crystals, books, stones, or objects adorned in neutral tones of soft brown and ochre. Where does earth reside within you? What part of your body does it represent?
- *Water*: An element related to emotions, fluids, and unconscious life. You can represent water with aquariums, fountains, water containers, or blue objects. Where does water reside within you? What part of your body does it represent?
- *Metal*: An element that unites everything, yet also brings focus and order. Consider incorporating metallic elements into your space—silver, shiny objects or metallic accents. Where does metal reside within you? What part of your body does it represent?

Ask yourself, observe, wait for the ideas to bloom, let the fusion of the elements happen naturally while you surrender to the unifying power of the night, when silence and darkness reign. Visualize your form: your body composed of all the elements, shedding what no longer serves it, so that chi renews itself with each breath.

☆ RITUAL 9. IN LOVE WITH YOUR HOUSE

1. Imagine your body as a house and the moment before sleep as an invitation to explore its depths.
2. Where are your walls? Where is the ceiling? Where do you place the pipes, the kitchen, and the bathroom?
3. Envision potential renovations. Are there areas that require repair, or perhaps even a complete redesign?
4. Do you feel the need to rearrange, recycle, or change something? Visualize your being wrapped in sheets and pillows in total relaxation, knowing that the night immersion will give you unexpected answers.

5. Activate your breath to accompany you, and then become your own architect. You can visualize the internal organs moving, without your intervention, to keep you alive: your precise and precious heartbeat.
6. Just like when you clean your house or room, choose, before entering the intangible zone of sleep, an idea or thought that paralyzes you. Identify it as clearly as possible and, consciously, decide to replace it with one of high vibration. Do this ritual every night and record any visions and insights that may emerge in your dreams.

Purpose and How to Use It

Paintings and movies often portray us as housewives—the hearth keepers, the guardians of walls and ceilings. We tend the fire in the stove, fill the pots, ensure spotless bathrooms and tidy beds. This societal role clings even to the most rebellious women—a nagging sense that true femininity demands complete devotion to the home. Yet, there is always something deep down: a lingering whisper that tells us we haven't fully embraced our domestic duty as mistress and lady of the house.

This dynamic extends to the bedroom, mirrored in the contractual obligation to sleep with one's partner every night, without the option to choose. This deeply ingrained expectation, woven into the fabric of societal norms, can make the idea of even one night alone a seemingly radical act of rebellion for many women.

In that physical and energetic jumble that takes place when you share your bed every night, the possibility of loving your body as your home fades away. You are constantly conditioned by the presence of another person—their desires, thoughts, energy, and dreams. The influence of energy transmission and of visible and invisible fluids cannot be stopped at the moment of deep sleep; on the contrary, it is sharpened by the vulnerability of the body and mind in the state of relaxation. Reclaiming a sense of sole ownership over your body can feel almost fantastical.

The time has come to love your own home, the one you inhabit, the temple that takes you from one place to another: the bones, tissues, flesh, and muscles that move in perfect coordination so that you are alive and present.

An inner sanctum, unknown to doctors, unmentioned in schools, ignored by family systems, and merely skimmed by psychologists: the internal home.

Within dwells the enigmatic essence and a perfect anatomy woven with powerful points that ignite pleasure, illuminate your path, and manifest your desires: it is the house where the soul acts out its earthly moments.

☆ RITUAL 10. LET YOUR TONGUE LOOSE AND DROOL WITHOUT RESTRICTIONS

The following ritual will make you a true housewife and mistress of the bed. I recommend its use at night for both the hygiene of the body and for better sleep.

1. Sitting on your bed before sleep, breathe, close your mouth, and use your nose to inhale and exhale. Now swallow saliva. Feel the movements of your mouth and throat as you swallow.
2. Feel your tongue in your mouth and run it over the inside of your cheeks, the entire palate, and under your teeth, slowly.
3. Swallow saliva again and notice if there are any changes from the first moment, when you started the ritual, to this point at which you have become aware of your mouth. Consciously, begin to bring your tongue to the roof of your mouth, curving it slightly so that it reaches the base of the two front teeth while you continue breathing. Then move it back a little more until it touches the center of the palate. As you do this, visualize how the back of your mouth opens, how the uvula moves, and how the entrance to your throat is cleared and free of obstacles, knots, and ready to express what you want without fear or prejudice.
4. Do this every night when you are alone to prepare your unconscious realm for a sidereal journey during slumber.

Purpose and How to Use It

The tongue, vital for digestion, the strongest muscle in your body, is attached at the back to the epiglottis and the hyoid bone, which connects to the thyroid and parathyroid glands. The tongue, with its taste receptors on the palate, is responsible for enunciating your words, as a bridge with the throat that unites the heart and the head. A tense tongue stifles the voice; if your voice falters, you won't be understood.

Rooted in ancient yogic traditions, this ritual guides you in harnessing powerful energy closures. The position of the tongue on the palate is called *jiva bandha* and refers to the physical closures of certain areas of the body that activate energy in order to ignite the flow of vital energy. Jiva bandha promotes flexibility of the frenulum of the tongue, expands the oral cavity, prevents jaw tension, and activates the parasympathetic system (the part of the nervous system that moderates anxiety and calms the brain and internal organs), producing saliva and enhancing mental focus.

Try to do this internal gesture with your tongue and palate whenever you remember, and notice what happens as a result in the tone of your thoughts and what you feel compelled to say. Observe how this practice enhances your ability to speak clearly, say the right thing, be heard, and gain respect for what you propose. Remember that everything starts within you and, as an entrepreneur of your own freedom, these mystical closures increase your frequency and electromagnetic field, attracting positive outcomes effortlessly and with grace.

From the moment of birth, our tongue serves as a primary tool: a conduit for sucking, a canvas for taste, and a powerful instrument of speech. Words, for better or worse, become the tongue's greatest wonder, capable of both exquisite expression and regrettable slips.

The very word *lingua* (Latin for tongue) hints at its deeper connection to language. Preparing your tongue before sleeping alone is one of the most powerful practices you can do on a spiritual level.

By night, you program your tongue—the sole internal organ to venture beyond the body—to connect with high-vibration energy.

This nocturnal ritual empowers your speech during the day, transforming how you express your truth—the words you choose, the delivery, and the very tone that carries your message.

Under the cloak of night, this practice and the understanding of what the tongue means as a sexual, sensual, and mystical territory will allow you to savor your fantasies, salivate, drool, and leave traces of your divine being wherever you please, without anyone holding you back, commenting, or criticizing.

☆ RITUAL 11. THE CEREBRAL PATHWAYS

1. Before placing your head on the pillow, gently massage your temples with the index fingers of each hand. Apply a steady, moderate pressure, avoiding excessive force while maintaining physical contact.

2. Move your fingers in a clockwise direction, followed by a counterclockwise motion. Repeat this movement fifteen times for each side, keeping your fingers on your temples throughout. As you perform the massage, pay attention to any physical or emotional sensations that arise. Once you have finished, lie down and close your eyes. Focus on the sounds you hear, allowing them to wash over you.

3. Now, adjust the position of your fingers: place just one index finger between your eyebrows, and repeat the same massage technique, moving in both clockwise and counterclockwise directions. Maintain a consistent yet gentle pressure, ensuring it's neither too intense nor too light.

4. Finally, create a mudra (a symbolic hand gesture) by placing your thumbs on your temples and your index fingers between your eyebrows, as if forming a halo. Breathe deeply, feeling the connection between these two points.

5. At this stage, focus on calming your breath. Inhale and exhale gently, bringing awareness to your abdomen in order to deepen your breath beyond the chest.

Purpose and How to Use It

We spend a third of our lives sleeping, and the quality of this rest is as essential as drinking water or eating. During sleep, a cascade of communication occurs between neurons that release toxins accumulated during wakefulness from the brain and body.

Therefore, this detoxification effect must be carried out meticulously every night. When entering sleep without company, the potential for this cleansing is enhanced, as the subjective and subtle interventions of the other person's brain waves do not interrupt this extraordinary individual process.

The temples are a junction where four cranial bones converge: the frontal, parietal, temporal, and sphenoid bones. They are located on the sides of the head, above the eye, between the forehead and the ear. The temporal muscle covers this area and is used during chewing.

This area isn't called a "temple" for no reason. Touching the acupressure point here honors that sacred space. It's no coincidence that gray hair often appears first in this area, a symbolic reminder of the knowledge and maturity it represents.

During this ritual, your touch transcends mere massage. By stimulating the temporal vein near your temple, you directly influence the cerebral cortex. Through the temples, you can clearly feel the beating of your heart, as they are not covered by a bone. This area, naturally sensitive to touch, is often where you place your fingers unconsciously when seeking focus. Use it to your advantage during the night to produce greater blood flow to the brain and achieve a higher vibration in your dreams.

By gently touching the space between your eyebrows, you gain direct access to the inner structures of your brain, including the pineal gland. This gland is responsible for producing melatonin—a key hormone in regulating your circadian rhythms and ensuring they are in perfect balance.

This ritual ignites a connection to your innate wisdom, guiding your inner eye toward a state of perfect balance. As you honor the rhythms of the night, undisturbed by external distractions, you awaken your auditory senses, emulating the nocturnal guardians of the forest—the owls and wolves. In this process, you transform into a woman of profound sensitivity and emotional power.

Ask yourself: What does the night sound like? What difference do you perceive in the sounds compared to those of the day? What emotions arise? What memories flood in? Sleep has an effect on the entire body on various levels—molecular, energetic, intellectual functions, alertness, and mood. Sleep helps to improve reflexes, enhance focus, and promote mindfulness.

Sleep impacts body tissues, hormones, growth, the immune system, and cardiovascular health. Tuning in to imperceptible sounds sharpens your mindfulness to a maximum point. By becoming receptive to distant or internal whispers, you make yourself available to hear the truths, mysteries, and questions that ignite your inner fire, spark your heart, and illuminate your own life and the lives of others.

Awaken to the messages you receive within your dreams. Your attuned awareness will retain them, empowering your waking life. Through the ritual, seek guidance and enlightenment; your wise inner teachers will speak directly to your heart.

☆ RITUAL 12. ONLY YOU CAN DO IT

1. Take advantage of those moments in bed before closing your eyes—that space where the light of consciousness begins to dim—to start this practice. Whether it's a change you desire, a daunting project you are undertaking, a limiting belief you hold, or a difficult situation you face, start by stating your name, then declare, "Only you can do it." For example: "Cynthia, only you can do it."
2. Repeat, "Only you can do it."
3. Once more, "Only you can do it."
4. In bed, when you are in your spiritual retreat, you can program anything you want to happen during the day by implanting a

magical and sacred word or phrase. Each of the letters, put together, generate an infallible vibrational combination that enters your unconscious world during sleep.

5. At night, before bed, repeat "only you can do it" three times to seal this pact of coexistence with yourself, and you will have brilliant results in the glory of your waking life.

Purpose and How to Use It

By speaking to yourself in the second person, many things happen in the biochemistry of your brain and in the space of emotions—you reframe your internal dialogue and listen, with perspective, to your wisest and most prolific voice guiding you on the right path.

If you've never tried it before, now is the time. Try speaking to yourself in the second person as a concrete and powerful meditation, as a reminder of the possibility of accessing the different subtle bodies that make up your person.

Beyond your physical form, a multitude of energy layers exist within and around you, ever-present companions. In the tradition of kundalini yoga these are understood as ten distinct bodies, each occupying a unique space and level of being.

Sufi masters, adherents of a mystical tradition rooted in Islam, assert that ten thousand universes manifested in energy lie close to our very flesh and bones. Yogis, on the other hand, speak of chakras—energy wheels aligned along the spine—and seventy-two thousand *nadis*—additional energy channels that circulate through the bloodstream.

When you use your voice to name yourself in the second person, you immediately open access to those other energies, electromagnetic fields, angelic presences, higher guides, and awakened messengers who are waiting to be summoned by you.

Like all spiritual practices, this one thrives on consistency. Start doing it every day, two or three times—especially when you need to get back on track, focus, "ground yourself," or find a space of calm and understanding, or when you are clouded by dark and debilitating thoughts, draining emotions, forces of insurmountable obstacles, mental movies of catastrophes, or the crippling "I can't." In these instances, the force of second-person language empowers you to finally put an end to these internal conflicts once and for all:

- Shatter limiting beliefs.
- Release thoughts of suffering and scarcity.
- Break free from the grip of lack.
- Sever ancestral contracts that bind you to a life of suffering.
- Silence the inner critic that sabotages joy and pleasure. Be wary of phrases like: "I can't afford it," "I can't pay for it," "I don't have the budget," "I don't have the time," "I don't know if I can," "My finances won't allow it," "I'm not qualified," "I won't be able to continue," and "I don't have the resources."

It's time to eradicate these self-limiting beliefs. We must replace "I can't" and "I don't" with the empowering language of possibility.

By embracing this ritual, you can effectively quell the anxiety stirred by foreboding thoughts of the future, revealing an uncharted realm that invites you to explore and become intimately acquainted with its depths.

This is the realm of loving and practical limits, where nothing and no one determines your decisions, where you listen to the intelligence of your heart in all its expansion, and you are the captain of your destiny and your desires. In this space, you program your dreams to come true in the waking state.

☆ RITUAL 13. LIBERATION OF BEINGS

1. With conscious intention and unwavering motivation, set your mind on liberating animals. I suggest performing this ritual in the hours or moments before bed, making it one of your last conscious acts of the day. This serves as a means of programming your subconscious as you prepare for rest.
2. You may liberate insects or animals that you cross paths with, either within your home or in the outside world, intentionally setting them free. A cockroach you spare, a fly you guide

through the open door, an ant you allow to wander freely. As you release them, evoke your deepest desire for their liberation. Direct your consciousness, focusing on each step of this process.

3. Establish a connection with these beings through the rhythm of your heart and breath. Observe them with an open mind, letting go of judgment and prejudice. Cultivate new emotions toward them, replacing feelings of disgust with compassion; rejection with acceptance. Remember, they are alive and, like you, desire happiness.
4. Prepare to release them, to grant them their freedom. Begin with a prayer or invocation, asking for their joy and liberation. Intentionally weave your own liberation into this act. May this freedom symbolize the release of outdated and useless ideas within yourself. Embrace the ritual's power—a symbolic cleansing for your body and mind, freeing you from stagnation and empowering your growth and evolution.
5. Gently blow toward the creature (ant, cockroach, fly, etc.), offering them your blessing accompanied by a silent prayer.
6. Set them free while you breathe and connect.

Purpose and How to Use It

Animal liberation is a Buddhist practice, powerful in its limitless expansion and transformative symbolism.

Releasing sentient beings from captivity with conscious intention has a profound and comprehensive impact. This act transforms the brain, fostering new neural connections as centuries of mechanical habits are broken, granting a new perspective on the interconnection of all beings.

Free an insect—from the fly struggling in a glass to the cockroach traversing your home, the buzzing mosquito, or the bee that you are about to step on. Consider rescuing abandoned dogs or cats, extending care and putting forth every effort to find them a loving home.

This is a conscious action with profound implications—particularly for cultivating positive emotions before sleep. It aims to foster the idea that all life is sacred—from the insect you despise, or the rat that repels you, to the spider that claims your ceiling as its home, or the ants that raid your plants. Every life is sacred.

From the tiniest larvae to the majestic whales, all sentient beings, including the diverse human species, are interconnected parts of a grand whole. Without each of these precious components, the intricate tapestry of life would be incomplete.

By freeing captive animals, I free myself and other humans who are physically or emotionally in captivity.

By releasing birds from their cages, I break my chains.

By pulling a beetle out of a puddle, I release myself from my permanent state of drowning.

I see and recognize the temporality of everything in that instant when I decide to save, release, let go. When I do this, I start to generate new images and connections in my mind: images of glory and relief, of joy and fluidity.

When I rescue a sentient being, I am saving myself, uncovering my mind, and igniting the heart of the world.

Starting today, cultivate the intention that, whenever possible and within your means, you may serve as an instrument of liberation. In the realm of your dreams, in the pleasure of the bed solely for yourself, this conscious act will have a profound impact on all the dimensions you traverse in your dreams. In this way, you will find many answers to questions that have been swirling in your mind for a long time.

☆ RITUAL 14. GUARDIANS OF THE NIGHT

1. Adorn your home with fresh flowers, either purchased or handpicked. Choose vibrant, abundant blooms that exude vitality and place them beside your bed.
2. The more colors you incorporate, the more powerful the nightly kaleidoscope of this ritual will be in filling your dreamscape with floral splendor.
3. Before retiring for the night, arrange the flowers in a circular mandala (a geometric figure representing the universe in

Hindu and Buddhist symbolism) on your bed. You can place them directly on the sheets or on a towel to protect your sleeping area.

4. The number of flowers is not as important as their orderly arrangement. Focus on creating a harmonious circle and pay attention to the interplay of shapes and colors.
5. Each flower represents your desires, visions, and aspirations. As you arrange them, engage in a meditative movement, naming each flower and anticipating fragrant dreams.
6. Perform your ceremony in honor of beauty as the perfume and colors begin to permeate your mattress, sheets, and the surrounding atmosphere.
7. Gaze upon the flowers, then close your eyes, imprinting their image on your mind. Repeat this practice several times, until it becomes your own.
8. When you are ready to sleep, place the flowers beside your bed as an offering for the night to come. They will serve as guardians of your dreams.

Purpose and How to Use It

In subtlety lies profound strength. Flowers are the ultimate embodiment of this combination. Upon close observation they never cease to amaze, for they are miniature worlds unto themselves. Each of their petals and everything that surrounds them, spreading out in seemingly fragile beauty, holds, in reality, the pure strength of the elemental world.

When you create these floral mandalas, the unconscious mind unexpectedly opens up and, through it, you connect directly with the plant kingdom, which is also part of your identity.

Your mandala's emanations are an offering to yourself. You deserve to surround yourself with beauty, plant flowers in your path, give yourself flowers as a gift. They are part of your essence—delicate and strong, always sharing beauty.

That communal circular form leaves impressions on your mind, so that during the night your lucid dreams are in technicolor and you can see ranges of tones that the human eye in the daytime could never capture.

You will craft a path of flowers before drifting off to sleep that will undoubtedly transport you to enchanting realms as you ascend in the four-legged spaceship of your bed.

Upon waking, I encourage you to surrender these blossoms to the earth or in the water (if a lake, river, or ocean lies within your reach). Returning them to the earth will allow their abundance to manifest in your life whenever you call upon them.

Honor the flowers on your nocturnal and diurnal journeys.

CHAPTER THREE

MANTRAS OF EMPOWERMENT

Whether you are familiar with mantras or these sounds are new to you, this chapter and its sacred repetitions will transmute your mind and emotions, carrying you toward a calm and clearer place. Without a doubt, mantras are an essential preparation for bedtime. By incorporating them into your life, your entire system will feel peace and harmony when you close your eyes and surrender to rest in the dream world.

Mantra is a Sanskrit word composed of two parts: *manas*, meaning "the mind or thought," and *tra*, which is the vehicle. Mantra is literally the vehicle of the mind or the transport that takes us beyond our established ideas.

In Buddhism and Hinduism (as well as other spiritual paths), reciting mantras is considered the best way to protect the mind. The mantra's high power resides in its sound and its vibrations, rather than the meaning of the words that are repeated.

Singing these sounds unleashes a cascade of scientifically proven benefits in the body, awakening the heart's intelligence and organizing the brain. Mantras are highly healing, powerfully expanding, limitless in their ancestral medicine, and wonderful for opening the head and throat before venturing into the mysterious night.

For this chapter, I have chosen mantras that are essential to me—that have accompanied me always, have saved my life and my mind, that are there in moments of anguish or joy. Simply repeating them brings attention to the breath and heartbeat, creates heart-brain synchrony, and balances the entire hormonal system. In the throat, the resonance of the mantra is sacred, and the vibration it produces is unparalleled to anything else you could say. By repeating it, you bless your voice, generate your own rhythm, and focus your attention on the sacred. Each time your tongue touches the upper palate, emitting these sounds, you activate spaces of your higher centers—enlightening the crystals of your pineal gland, which begin to expand your ideas and beliefs.

A mantra is a poem that passes through your entire body and influences your vagus nerve. The moment you begin to repeat it, from your throat to all your vital organs, you create an unexpected alchemy that becomes your reservoir of health and activates your high immune system.

Before bed, repeat them; let them sink into the folds of your brain, let them flow through your veins, let your heart pump them to the tips of your toes and back, circulating freely through all your sacred spaces. Here I will share some Tibetan, Arabic, Hebrew, Lakota, and Sanskrit mantras. They are my unparalleled treasures, and they will help you through your journey of dreams. You can ask for your own special sound—the one that vibrates and resonates most deeply with your soul.

I also recommend that you write them down to keep them handy for when you need them. You can even put them under your pillow or mattress so that their emanations reach you all the time. They will become the vehicle for your mind to reach a higher and more elevated state.

☆ RITUAL 15. *GAM ZU L'TOVAH* (PRONOUNCED GAM-ZOO-LE-TOH-VAH)

1. Settle into your bed before sleep and focus on your body. If thoughts arise, let them pass. Breathe and begin repeating this mantra. Feel the power of the vibrations and notice what you are feeling and what emotions come up when you say these words.
2. At this time, bring your right hand to your left wrist to take your pulse. Place your index and middle fingers on the area of the veins and feel how, while repeating this Hebrew mantra, a journey of union begins between your words and your heartbeat.
3. Continue repeating *Gam Zu L'Tovah* until you feel your breath calm completely. Then, incorporate a visualization of gratitude into your repetition. Bring to mind three specific things you are grateful for—they can be people, situations, or moments. Try to imagine them with the greatest detail, as if you could touch them.
4. Now, give thanks in advance. Include in these visualizations the projects and dreams you have for the future, as if they were happening right now, as if they had materialized at this moment.
5. Continue breathing in the energy of Gam Zu L'Tovah and maintain your repetition for at least three minutes, so that the effect of these words opens new channels and neuronal interconnection. Use a timer to make sure you do it for the allotted time. When you have finished, take a deep breath, close your eyes, and surrender to a magnificent sleep.

Purpose and How to Use It

"Everything happens for a reason," "This too shall serve a higher purpose," "Unwavering faith in the process," "Complete trust in the flow of things," "Every experience holds a valuable lesson."

These could be some ways to interpret and translate the Hebrew phrase *Gam Zu L'Tova*. This phrase appears in the Talmud and contains a powerful healing technology in each of its letters.

In Jewish mysticism, Hebrew letters contain a divine seal and are considered to be gateways to the celestial world. When studied, they reveal secrets of the cosmos. Knowing and pronouncing them connects us directly to our intuition and supports our highest healing and clairvoyant powers.

Repeating this mantra produces a high-quality vibration. It instantly works as a balm against negativity and anxiety. If we let go and trust that what seems dark and sinister also has a purpose, then the division between good and bad, black and white, and hard and soft is integrated.

The sharp edges of our mind become polished, and we begin to gradually step back from the precarious ledge that dominates our lives—always on the edge of the precipice, dangerously bordering the unstable terrain of crises, oscillating wildly between fleeting triumphs and crushing defeats.

Let the power of Gam Zu L'Tovah shine in your meditation and daily practice, and then you can surrender, integrate, and understand that events, emotions, thoughts, successes, and mistakes always hold something intrinsically good.

Ultimately, everything teaches us something. Every experience is a learning opportunity. When these Hebrew words come out of our mouths, we ascend to a high-scale vibrational level that amplifies understanding and illuminates our path.

On a physical level, in the body, this phrase resonates throughout its entirety due to the power of the Hebrew letters. Each letter has multiple possibilities for interpretation. They are complete symbols formed by numerology, astrology, sacred geometry, and kabbalah to help us navigate our opinions about what is right and what is wrong.

On an emotional level, these words, their letters, and the sound they produce have a high vibration that corresponds to a coherent resonance between the heartbeat, the heart's rhythm, and our brain waves. They provide immediate relief from neurosis and, above all, from ruminating, obsessive, and endless thoughts that only bring suffering and exhaustion.

It is excellent to pronounce before sleeping and to use as a blessing at the same time.

☆ RITUAL 16. *LOKAH SAMASTHA SUKHINO BHAVANTHU* (PRONOUNCED AS WRITTEN)

1. Settle your head on your pillow, feeling your body relax into the bed. As you breathe, repeat the mantra, gradually incorporating each word until the sound becomes familiar to your ears. Don't worry if your pronunciation isn't perfect; it is your connection with the sounds that matters.
2. As you repeat the mantra, let your awareness expand to encompass the living beings around you. Feel their presence and honor their existence. Allow the experience to unfold organically, embracing the images and emotions that arise within you.
3. Honor the unseen multitudes that dwell within you; the bacteria and microbes form a vibrant ecosystem. Extend this respect to those beyond, in all their diverse forms. As you repeat this mantra, visualize yourself enveloped in a radiant aura of self-love—a vital force for your wellbeing.
4. Include your family, friends, neighbors, coworkers, acquaintances, and strangers. Include all the humans around you, even those who are no longer here—those who have departed and whom you carry in your heart.
5. Expand your vision from the smallest to the largest until you can encompass all living beings on this planet and in the galaxies.
6. As you visualize, maintain awareness of your heartbeat. Let the mantra flow on your lips, and notice any subtle shifts in your heart's rhythm or the quality of your experience.
7. As you prepare for sleep, culminate the ritual by caressing your entire body in a gesture of gratitude. Honor your living being and the service you provide to the world. You are the heart of this mantra and ritual: cherish your existence, your life force, and your potential for growth as you expand your light.

Purpose and How to Use It

This Sanskrit mantra resounds with profound clarity: "May all beings, in every realm, find happiness and freedom." As you chant or recite these sacred words, your heart resonates in harmony with the heartbeat of the universe. No being is excluded; all receive the blessings of your recitation: those within you—the trillions of organisms sustaining your digestive system, the guardians of your skin's defense against infection, the microscopic microbes and bacteria essential for your balanced health—even the sentient beings beyond your physical form, for everything around you possesses spirit and life—even the seemingly inanimate, like a mineral.

This potent mantra transcends the confines of self and ego, expanding your worldview and triggering a ripple effect that impacts all that surrounds you. As you recite it, it erases preconceived notions about whom to love and whom not to love, and whom to wish well upon and whom not. It places all beings on equal footing, elevating you to the same level as every living, breathing creature. A mosquito is no less than a human; all are worthy of receiving the emanations of this powerful mantra.

To break down its Sanskrit meaning, *Lokah* signifies "the world"—not just our earthly realm but the vast expanse of all universes. *Samastah* means "the whole." *Sukhino* is "happiness." *Bhavantu* means "may all." As you whisper this mantra before sleep, you reach a peace agreement with your ruminating and recurring mental noises, allowing seamless transition into the realm of dreams, where you commune with the entirety of existence. Install it as a nightly ritual, so that you can record what happens while you sleep alone, and feel the sacred presence that permeates all that surrounds you, a presence you have lovingly blessed.

☆ RITUAL 17. *SA TA NA MA*

1. Seated on your bed, you will use the ancestral strength and power of your hands to perform this ritual. Use both hands in order for the ritual's effect to be complete and balanced throughout your entire organism. Before sleeping, start off

by touching your thumb with your index finger and saying *Sa*, which means birth, or the origin of everything.
2. Then, touch your thumb with your middle finger saying *Ta*— life and its creative manifestation.
3. Without losing your rhythm, touch your thumb with your ring finger saying *Na*, or death and transformation.
4. Finally, touch your thumb with your little finger saying *Ma*— rebirth, regeneration, and conscious presence of infinite magnificence.
5. Do it with both hands at the same time while you breathe and reap the fruits of the perfect cycles that nourish your life.
6. First, repeat *Sa Ta Na Ma* aloud for one minute, then continue in a whisper for another minute, and, finally, repeat it mentally. Record what happens when you listen to yourself, when your voice diminishes, and when it only resonates within you. Then surrender to sleep, with the certainty that the perfect cycle will occur while you rest.

Purpose and How to Use It

Every process manifests in a circular fashion. There is no definitive beginning or end, for everything that creates us, everything we are, depends on other things, on other factors. Not a single manifestation in this world exists independently: everything is inextricably linked as part of an eternal and ascending cycle. Consider anything you use, eat, consume, or employ; if you break down its components, you'll clearly recognize that all of its elements depend on each other, that they function in a cycle, and that the ritual of Sa Ta Na Ma is present in every part of your existence:

- In the way you breathe, in the cycles of your inhalation and exhalation.
- The cycles of nature with its seasons.
- The processes of plants and insects.
- Everything is perfectly aligned, interconnected with every other thing in a spiral.

The manifestations of sentient beings, the workings of the invisible planes, even the intricate dance of internal biological processes—all are woven together in a tapestry of infinitesimal detail.

Everything that exists follows the cycle of Sa Ta Na Ma, birth, life, death, and rebirth—a rhythm echoed in everything, including our sleep. As you drift off alone in bed, consider this mantra as you embark on your mystical night's journey. Throughout your slumber, even as your consciousness travels to unseen realms, you traverse the cycle's entirety. Each night, you unknowingly enact this cycle hundreds of times. By harnessing this experience upon waking, you rise with a renewed sense of awareness—you are both a thread in the cosmic tapestry and a being of infinite freedom, forever connected yet uniquely detached.

In Sanskrit, the individual syllables are the linguistic root of *Sat Nam*, "my true essence" or "my true identity."

- *Sa* represents birth and the beginning of the entire cosmos.
- *Ta* signifies life, existence, and manifested creativity.
- *Na* symbolizes death and transformation.
- *Ma* represents rebirth, regeneration, and the experience of infinite bliss.

Together, Sa Ta Na Ma encapsulates the endless cycle of birth, growth, death, and rebirth.

In my personal yoga and meditation practice, this is one of my favorite mantras because it detaches me from expectations, places me on the observer's throne, and simultaneously induces a hypnotic effect of vibrational upliftment.

When repeating this mantra, strive for mindfulness and full attention—not only on the finger movements with each syllable, but also on the position of your tongue inside your mouth as you pronounce each part. When you say *Sa*, your tongue should remain down, touching your lower teeth, allowing air to flow freely. When you say *Ta* and *Na*, place the tip of your tongue upward, touching the point where the palate begins between your front teeth. Then say *Ma*, with your tongue down again, just like when you started. By doing this, the tongue movements activate energy points and body meridians that directly influence the proper functioning of the pineal gland, responsible for producing melatonin, a vital hormone for rest and for the homeostatic balance of your body.

Your circadian rhythms will be perfect; your sleep will be deep and restorative, leaving you energized and focused throughout the day. No more midday slumps! This newfound rhythm will allow you to effortlessly flow through your waking hours, while ensuring a peaceful night's rest.

By repeating these syllables, the combination of sounds and movements will allow any cycle you are going through to flow gracefully. Observe how the pronunciation of these high vibrations reverberate in your mouth, generating a current of positive energy throughout your body. This act ignites your inner luminescence, fostering protection against negativity and softening the rigidity of crisis reactions. With newfound awareness of the cyclical nature of existence, endings lose their dramatic weight, replaced by the knowledge of inevitable rebirth. As the moon ascends, embark on your nocturnal journey, empowered by this ritual and mantra to illuminate your path, clear obstacles, and find fulfillment.

☆ **RITUAL 18. *OM MANI PADME HUM***

1. Settle into bed. Repeat this sacred six-syllable mantra, touching different parts of your body as you do so. It is best done before sleep.
2. When you say *Om*, touch your forehead with the fingers of your right hand, trying to feel the space between your eyebrows and the vibration that occurs there.
3. When you say *Ma*, touch your throat area and feel the vibration of this sound in your neck.
4. When you say *Ni*, touch your heart, feeling your heartbeat.
5. When you say *Pad*, touch the pit of your stomach; that space between your ribs, in the solar plexus.

6. When you say *Me*, bring your fingers below your navel, activating the resonance in the space of your uterine altar.
7. When you say *Hum*, bring both hands to your lower back, around the kidneys, while extending the sound of the syllable to that area.
8. Try to do at least three rounds of this circuit and the movements that accompany each syllable. If you can, do it with your eyes closed, visualizing each of the activated parts with the image of a lotus flower growing in your body. When you complete the three rounds of the circuit, you can surrender to sleep.

Purpose and How to Use It

Chanting this mantra awakens something utterly pure and magical within you, for each syllable offers a tribute to the lotus flower's symbolism, drawing you closer to your own inner jewel. Like this magnificent bloom, beauty can be born even from darkness and adversity. The lotus, brimming with healing power, emerges immaculate from stagnant waters—a testament to the enduring potential for spiritual evolution that resides within us all.

When you repeat this mantra, its benefits ripple outward, touching not only you but those around you. By repeating it before drifting off to sleep, you receive virtues, your wisdom grows, and this practice becomes a gentle guide, calming the mind and opening the heart.

The mantra consists of six syllables, each representing a form of perfection, a vehicle to exalt your inner yearning. By repeating it as part of your preparation for the lucid dream journey, you cleanse your subtle channels and balance key areas of your body.

The third eye, throat, heart, stomach, uterus, and kidneys resonate with each of these syllables, like a bath of internal and external purification, as each repetition balances mental disturbances, negativity, and mental noise. I'll break down the meaning of each syllable so that each time you repeat the mantra, you may feel the shift toward emotional harmony.

CHAPTER THREE ⭐ MANTRAS OF EMPOWERMENT

- *Om* is the sound of generosity. It dissolves ego pride. Om resonates on the forehead, melting glaciers of stagnant ideas.
- *Ma* is the sound that represents ethical behavior and the dissolution of jealousy. Ma opens up proper and loving communication in the throat.
- *Ni* is the sound that represents patience and dissolves excessive passion and desire, compulsions, and addictions toward different things or people. You can hear Ni vibrating in the center of the heart while you activate calm in each beat.
- *Pad* is the sound that represents diligence, willingness, and openness of ideas; it dissolves ignorance and prejudice. Pad is situated in the pit of the stomach, recognizing the diaphragm muscle activating paralyzed digestive processes.
- *Me* is the sound that represents renunciation and dissolves possessiveness and greed, allowing for an observation of your own tendencies, without judgment and with great self-respect. By placing your hands on your lower abdomen, on your uterus, you recognize your power center and ignite the altar of creativity and the gestation of ideas and projects that live in this area of your body.
- *Hum* is the sound that represents wisdom and dissolves aggression, hatred, anger, and rage. Unrestrained and violent reactions are transmuted; you are no longer a tangle of nerves and anger, but a conscious woman who can manage her emotions from a new, revolutionary place. The kidneys are responsible for purifying and expelling what does not serve you.

After completing three rounds of movement and sound, I recommend that you remain silent for a moment, breathing, feeling the impact of these syllables and your hands on your body. Visualize your organism being reborn, flourishing, wide open, like a lotus flower, into the world of your dreams. This mantra is a very powerful catalyst for lucid dreaming, based on the image of the flower that is born from the mud with all its majestic beauty.

☆ RITUAL 19. NOOR

1. In a relaxed position, before sleep, ask for *noor* (this Arabic word, pronounced as it is read, means light). You can be seated or semireclined on your bed.
2. Imagine a beam of light descending from above, enveloping you completely. Feel its warmth illuminate you from all angles: front, back, and along your right and left sides.
3. Now, visualize the light within your being, your flesh, your blood...
4. Do the noor meditation by picturing how the luminosity surrounds you and, at the same time, springs from your centers and your being to expand into the world.
5. You no longer just ask and receive, but you are also a generator of light—creating and giving in an unending cycle.
6. Now, start sending light to everything around you. Imagine rays permeating even the seemingly impenetrable corners. For areas where the light seems to struggle, envision tiny cracks allowing a luminous essence to seep through. This practice can illuminate stagnant ideas, situations that feel stuck, or even physical or health challenges that require improvement.
7. Close your eyes and activate the noor mantra meditation, bathing your bed, pillows, sheets, and blankets with this luminous energy for the night journey, redefining daily routines and turning it into a work of art.

Purpose and How to Use It

To practice this mantra most effectively, repeat it ninety-nine times. In Sufism, the number ninety-nine holds special significance, representing the sacred names and divine qualities of the creator, which you can cultivate within yourself. Use a *mala* (Hindu prayer beads), *tasbih* (Muslim prayer beads), or a ninety-nine-bead rosary to keep track and maintain focus. As you recite *noor* (light) and touch each bead, envision its light filling you. If you lack these tools, repeat the mantra naturally, calling out to the light everywhere until you feel that the vision is instilled within you. You are now a transmitter of clarity—from the inside out—and you will melt away centuries of stagnant ideas and concepts, repeated habits, and behaviors that prevent you from evolving.

On my Sufi path (I have been practicing this spiritual path for thirty years) and in my evolution as a musician and composer, *zikr* has served as a powerful bridge to the divine in my life. Zikr, akin to *kirtan*, involves the uninterrupted repetition of high-vibrational words, a sacred chant. As the sounds resonate and take shape in your throat, a sublime experience unfolds: light seems to enter effortlessly with each uttered mantra.

Noor—one of the sacred names of the divine qualities of the Creator—lies within you as well. This radiant essence is not an external force, but an inherent quality of your soul, though invisible to the human eye. Through it, you emit iridescent beams that, when activated, make you more prone to an open mind and an unguarded heart.

As you awaken the mantra and repetition within yourself, your autonomic nervous system and your vagus nerve, passing through your throat, vocal cords, the beating of your heart, and your enteric brain (in the intestine) balance toward the intention that light will be victorious.

By invoking the mantra for all areas and cardinal points of your body, you are generating the mental and emotional disposition to activate this luminous shield and, when you enter the realm of night and dreams, it leads you into very deep states of discovery.

In Arabic, the word *noor* and the repetition *Ya al Noor* also carry connotations of illuminating, enlightening, filling with light, clarifying, revealing, making visible, bringing the invisible to the senses, and guiding others. These multifaceted aspects of the word serve you well when you need to clarify ideas and concepts or find answers in situations where messages seem encrypted or you encounter dark obstacles.

If you feel like there is no light at the end of the tunnel and that hope is waning, use this sacred mantra. Take advantage of the ritual to fill your magical nighttime carpet, your spiritual retreat in the dark, with light. Bring this mantra to the parts of the bed that receive your body and ask for lots of light while you sing it, directing yourself especially toward your pillow so that everything that happens during sleep will be as clear as crystal and you will wake up full of certainties.

☆ RITUAL 20. *AHO MITAKUYE OYASIN* (PRONOUNCED AS WRITTEN)

1. Stand in front of your bed, rub your hands together, and gently pass them over your body. Use this moment to create supreme consciousness and maximum gratitude for each of the parts that make you human. Then, enter your nighttime spaceship. Lie down and start breathing, visualizing your interconnection with everything. All is interdependent; nothing exists on its own.

2. To achieve this, embark on a journey of self-discovery, exploring the intricate tapestry of your being. Delve into the mineral, animal, vegetal, and human realms that reside within you. Unveil the essence of your spirit and soul, the forces that sustain your existence, as well as the elements: fire, air, water, earth—both tangible and intangible.

3. Explore the areas where air touches your body when you connect with your breath; the water element in your fluids (saliva, blood, mucus); the fire element in your stomach, the seat of digestion; and the earth represented by your bones. The surrounding universe, a harmonious whole, governs all with perfect balance.

4. Now, repeat this mantra, focusing your brain on the divine network to which you belong. Repeat the mantra mentally while remaining aware of your inhalation and exhalation.

5. Take your practice into your nighttime experience by incorporating this interconnection into everything: bed, pillow, room, the visible and invisible elements that surround you, and the whispers of your intuition. All is one, and you have a relationship with all.

CHAPTER THREE ✦ MANTRAS OF EMPOWERMENT

6. *Aho Mitakuye Oyasin.* Repeat this mantra in honor of all your relationships.

Purpose and How to Use It

Mitakuye Oyasin, a Lakota mantra translating to "all my relations," serves as a powerful blessing. It's an "amen" for the interconnected web of life, encompassing not just humans, but everything within and beyond you. The level of consciousness that this repetition produces is incomparable and unites you with forests and rivers, mountains and seas, stones and insects. It acknowledges the unbroken timeline of existence—honoring your ancestors, origins, and all that sustains you. The practice fosters a deep gratitude, opening you to a heightened sense of perception and appreciation for the richness of your life.

Your very presence here speaks volumes about the interconnectedness of all things. You are sustained by the bounty of the whole, a collective energy field sometimes referred to as *morphic resonance*, or the *morphological field*. This unified mental field operates on a planetary level, weaving us all together.

Does this mean that our thoughts create an invisible network that feeds back on itself? As the mantra says, I create a collective memory that encompasses absolutely everything; therefore, everything I think, do, and say has a profound impact on the rest of my relationships.

The morphogenetic field is a territory of memory where living species move, reflecting that we depend on absolutely everything to continue existing. When I modify the vibrational frequencies of thoughts at the community level, recognizing and honoring all my relationships, my electromagnetic capacity inevitably expands. Likewise, brain circuits that produce synchronicity and harmony are modified, guiding me away from chaos and disorder.

This mantra, or prayer, is one of supreme power. It becomes sweet on your tongue—transforming your brain and impacting the intelligence of your heart. With complete certainty, this mantra confirms that we do not exist without other relationships, that we are absolutely dependent on each other.

The Lakota prayer of this mantra goes as follows:

I give thanks for the opportunity to acknowledge you in this prayer.

To the mineral nation, which builds and sustains my bones and the foundation of all living experience, planets, and stars, I thank you.

To the plant nation, for the oxygen in every breath that sustains my organs and body and that gives me plants and medicinal herbs to heal myself, I thank you.

To the animal nation, which feeds me with its life and flesh and offers me loyal companionship on my life's journey, I thank you more than words can say.

To the human nation for the help, love, and friendship I receive, I thank you.

To the nation of spirits, to the Great Spirit who has carried light through the ages, for the gift of encounters and the beauty of taking the weight of the world off my shoulders, I thank you.

To the four winds of change and growth, I thank you.

You are my relationships, my family, without whom I would not be alive.

We are in the circle of life together, coexisting, codependent, and cocreating our destiny. No one is more important than another. All, part of the great mystery. Thank you for this life.

From now on, weave this grand ritual into the very fabric of your being. Let it infuse your every breath, guide your endeavors, and deepen your daily spiritual initiation. As you embark on your nightly journey, invite all your relations to join you. Here, what no longer serves you will gently detach, while blessings effortlessly flow into your life.

CHAPTER THREE ☆ MANTRAS OF EMPOWERMENT

☆ RITUAL 21. SOHAM

1. Lie down, relax, feel your body entering a state of calm and gratitude. As you inhale, draw out the syllable *So* on your breath, savoring the sound as it fills your mouth and mind.
2. With a deep exhale, release all the air from your lungs, uttering the word *Ham* as you do so. Let out a full sigh, emptying yourself completely, allowing the sound to fill the space around you.
3. Inhale: *So.*
4. Exhale: *Ham.*
5. Continue breathing with the syllables on your inhalation and exhalation as you relax more and more deeply.
6. As you continue breathing with both sounds, try to lower your breath to your abdomen, establishing diaphragmatic breathing. You can place your hand on your stomach to feel the movement of rising and falling, inflating and deflating, going from the thoracic space to the diaphragm muscle. By exhaling more deeply, you massage all your internal organs and release toxicity from the body.
7. Enter your presleep process with this mantra, preparing your mental and emotional territory for the interstellar journey you will take. You can repeat the mantra until you feel it becomes a lullaby that rocks you to sleep.

Purpose and How to Use It

SoHam is a Sanskrit word that means "I am," or "I am the universe." It serves to move you from a limited sense of self to a more complete, larger-scale conception of self, full of perspective and the certainty that you are part of something greater. Combining the syllables with the breath produces new cellular nourishment. The brain (membrane) of your cells receives the information that a more favorable environment is being created thanks to the high vibration of these words and unprecedented oxygenation. It is a great mantra for silencing the chatter of anxious thoughts. It enhances focus, guiding your mind toward goals and their successful completion.

These Sanskrit syllables bring the aroma of ancient spiritual traditions to an experience of the present moment, and each of these letters nourishes your biology with a high vibration.

Imagine your brain and heart aligning in perfect harmony, much like tuning a radio dial, until you find the desired frequency. By rhythmically repeating this mantra while focusing on your breath, you achieve this state of coherence.

Deepen your practice by visualizing the *So* as fresh forest greenery entering your body with each inhale. As you exhale, imagine the *Ham* as opening a reservoir within you, allowing you to receive new oxygen and shed all that no longer serves you.

You take and give back, inhale and exhale, *SoHam*.

As you continue with this mantra, you will begin to hear the sound everywhere, you will see how the entire universe accompanies you in your SoHam breathing. When it is time to sleep, breathing in time with this repetition will help you enter an almost hypnotic state that challenges any rebellion of the body to stay awake.

CHAPTER FOUR

DIVINE SENSUALITY

Your bed, this vessel for celestial slumber, is a portal to a realm of tranquility, solitude, and sensuality, a starry expanse mirroring the cosmos above. It is here, in this sanctuary of self-discovery, that you embark on an intimate exploration of your being—delving into the depths of your subtle bodies, the ethereal fluids that interweave with the matter that defines your humanity.

An ethereal sensuality that you explore at night, without company, and that produces a deep connection with your cosmogony, fills you with the certainty of being here and now and, at the same time, will reveal your beautiful vulnerability. Everything you do—the movements you make, the thoughts and sounds you emit—cultivates other bodily levels that are far from mundane noise. Rather, when integrated with the daytime experiences, your nighttime sensuality will make you float while you are awake.

The body in bed emits frequencies that, without interference, can expand much more, embracing other levels of consciousness within the miracle that you inhabit—your energetic anatomy, the use of your more tangible and subtle bodies, and the use of your fluids in an integral and waste-free way.

In treating illness, enlightened Tibetan Buddhist lamas advise their students on a unique self-healing method. Students are encouraged to anoint affected areas with their own saliva, while reciting sacred mantras to promote a faster recovery.

Imagine everything you can do with the manifestations of your body, from your menstruation to your sweat, integrating them divinely, without having to explain or ask anyone for permission. That is yours in total sovereignty; you do not have to hide or disguise, wash or perfume. In the entire expanse of your bed, you will find yourself.

You are pure energy. From your molecules to your emotions, your body is a major channel of biological processes that pass through your cells, flow in your blood, and navigate your breath. You are a compendium of vibrating information, and the sacred night alone gives you the great opportunity to explore it.

Let us advocate for a transcendental sensual experience that, each time it is activated, takes you beyond the senses. This practice empowers you to recognize your life-giving creative force with every breath—a spiritual and experiential sensuality where you infuse every touch with your soul and your spirit soars, silencing the mind, with sails unfurled, embraced by bliss. This luminous sensuality stems from the light within you, the microcrystals in your pineal gland that, when set in motion, generate a lighter electromagnetic field, elevating you beyond the ordinary constraints of existence.

This is a sensuality with its own language that reconnects all your intelligences and generates balance between light and darkness, enveloping your glands and hormones so that melatonin acts in supreme excellence.

In this chapter, you will go through rituals to awaken a sacred sensuality. Each ritual is connected with the seven universal principles with the seven chakras (and subtle bodies) and their master glands.

ASCENDING CHAKRAS EVERY SEVEN YEARS

For the purpose of this chapter on sensuality, it is essential to understand that, beyond the spiritual and esoteric view of chakras, or wheels of energy that are considered to connect the subtle with the corporeal at specific points of the body, these points have a direct relationship with the entire glandular system.

We evolve in seven-year cycles, with each stage focusing on a specific chakra and its corresponding area in the body. It is essential to understand that lower chakras vibrate at slower frequencies, while higher ones vibrate faster. This esoteric information regarding seven-year cycles and the evolution of consciousness in the body and spirit is fundamental to understanding the power that the possibility of spending your night alone holds.

Where are you currently on your chakra journey? How do your breath, thoughts, and words flow through these energy centers? While your age may influence the prominence of certain characteristics, emotions and experiences create a constant dance through all manifestations. The key takeaway is to approach this information with loving awareness, understanding how to cultivate your own potential for growth, freedom, and creativity, unbound by any specific stage. Solo sleep provides the perfect sanctuary for such exploration.

The first seven years of life center on the root chakra, *muladhara*. Here, the foundation of the personality is laid. We anchor to the earth, take those first steps, gain sphincter control, and develop a sense of self-worth ("I have the right to be here, to be listened to, and respected"). We transition from liquids to solids, begin to explore the world, and develop language and abstract thought. Esoteric philosophers, like Rudolf Steiner, posit that this stage is also marked by the symbolic shedding of baby teeth and the emergence of permanent ones, signifying the soul's full incarnation. The etheric forces that work in the child's organism begin to push out the baby teeth (which are inherited from the parents) and the permanent teeth make their appearance in a process that can last even until the end of the period corresponding to the next chakra—between 7 and 14 years old.

Between the ages of 7 and 14, individuals move on to the second chakra, located in the sacral area: *svadhishthana*, which is directly related to sexual energy, creativity, learning to identify and express emotions, prepuberty and puberty, and an extraordinary hormonal surge that affects all aspects of the body and spirit. A deeper understanding of sexuality begins to develop, and girls experience menstruation, undergoing some of their most significant rites of passage during this time. The second chakra corresponds to the testicles and ovaries, the gonads responsible for producing sex hormones. This marks the beginning of the expansion of individuality, the ability to express one's feelings, the development of intuition, and the expansion of consciousness.

Between the ages of 14 and 21, we move on to the solar plexus zone, *manipura*: leaving puberty and entering a stage of consolidation of more mystical existential searches. One begins to understand the self in relation to others, as the solar plexus reflects the bright center of the middle of the body. The vibrational levels of this space are higher and more subtle, resulting in the strong anchor to the earth and the personality gradually being left behind and beginning to feel the possibility of connection with the sacred, which resonates upward. This stage, which in the body is directly related to digestive processes, has a correlation at the spiritual level with the beginning of a consciousness that discriminates much more between what does and does not serve for the evolution of the being. Waste has to go out and nutrients have to stay. The center of power is transferred to personal power and intimate decisions about how to live dharma: the purpose of being here. This chakra is associated with the endocrine system, located in the pancreas.

From 21 to 28, we find ourselves evolving into the heart chakra, *anahata*: the power of the intelligence of the heart center, where more than forty thousand neurons beat, making this area of the body a complete brain. Many people find the love of their life in this stage, and others begin to love themselves with full consciousness and find appreciation for the planet. Gratitude for everything that happens takes on new dimensions and you begin to experience the possibility of breathing from the heart. The gland that governs this space is the thymus—the master gland of the immune system and, for some ancient traditions, the place where the soul resides. In this chakra I can fully reap the nourishment that I have given to spiritual life throughout all the previous years, understanding that the way I breathe and what I think alters and affects the way my heart beats. I take full responsibility for everything that happens to me and I can synchronize with absolute certainty my heart rate variability with my brain waves. The divine center of the heart is impregnated with high vibrations in words and intentions to generate an electromagnetic field full of joy and altruism. I can sit and contemplate life on the throne of emotions, knowing that I have entered a stage of adulthood in which I choose with whom and how I want to live.

From 28 to 35, we find ourselves moving on to the throat area, *vishuddha*: the word, communication; the conjunction of all the elements that combine to emit a powerful voice—your own voice, the one that says what you think and feel in a coherent and calm way, without hesitation, hoarseness, or aphonia. This chakra gives music and voice to what comes from the heart and is the last space that processes the coarsest elements of the physical world; from here on there is only spiritual ascension. When you live in this biological age, many of the adolescent issues have already been left behind. The prefrontal cortex is fully developed; therefore, decisions, ideas, and manifestations come from a calm and balanced space. Here is where you find your voice, untie the knots in your throat that have silenced you, and let your voice rise, unshackled and true. This chakra is related to the thyroid, which regulates body temperature, metabolism, and the development of nerve cells, among others. Likewise, the vagus nerve is a fundamental component of the biological balance of this chakra, since it directly touches the areas of the pharynx, larynx, vocal cords, thyroid, and parathyroid glands. By creating a propitious environment for calm breathing, with the precise use of the facial resonators and the proper handling of the vocal cords without tension, a nirvana of maturity full of joy and wisdom is reached.

From 35 to 42, you have ascended to higher areas: *ajna*, the chakra located in the third eye, between your eyebrows. Everything is governed by intuition, ancestral wisdom, synthesis of information, a place of illumination and epiphanies. You perfectly understand the synchronization between all your centers. This is where the pituitary gland (hypophysis) or master gland of the endocrine system is located. When you activate this zone, you produce a mystical awakening that is no longer related to your senses, but to the astral bodies (nonmaterial). In the field of biology, the main function of the pituitary gland is to produce hormones that regulate vital functions and processes such as metabolism, growth, sexual maturation, reproduction, and blood pressure, among others. All these functions correspond to spiritual understanding. It is in this age range that the being already knows deeply what his or her mission is and manifests all the means to carry it out.

From ages 42 to 49, you'll have reached the crown chakra: *sahasrara*, the final chapter of the seven-year cycle, related to spiritual awakening and elevated expansion. Intuition becomes tangible, and lucid dreams brimming with information become commonplace. The crown chakra is where the pineal gland resides, controlling the production of melatonin, which regulates the circadian sleep-wake cycle. It is the perfect terrain to experience your spiritual retreat by sleeping alone. Free from external disturbances of light or noise, you hold the power to control your environment and enter into a deep sleep, maximizing your pineal gland's potential.

Keep in mind that the pineal gland alters melatonin production according to the amount of light it perceives through the eye, which is why it is also called the "Eye of Horus." At this stage, you already know all the physical and emotional ups and downs that go through your body and it will be easy for you to establish a rigorous meditation and breathing practice. It is a great opportunity to connect with your guru, with the ascended masters, with angels and archangels.

BUT WHAT HAPPENS AFTER YOU TURN 49?

The time has come to ascend, to embark on or continue a spiritual revolution that transcends the realm of the senses. A crossroads lies before you—either you regress to an initial stage (the genital chakra) where you are moved by your sphincter impulses, where you stumble when you walk and feel like you are the center of the universe, just like a baby, or you decide to rise, grow, and ascend.

Imagine soaring upward, venturing into your intangible zone. This is where you can reclaim your body, the home of your unconscious mind. Open yourself to extraordinary perceptions and embrace the freedom to be unburdened by societal expectations. However, a regression to the root chakra is very common in men. It can manifest as reluctance to mature; this is why we often see older men seeking young women and dressing and acting like teenagers with a propensity for misogyny and melodrama. These behaviors represent a descent, a resistance to personal growth

The truth is that the choice to ascend and evolve is voluntary. It is your decision, your choice, but you must do so with full awareness, knowing that this implies total responsibility for everything you say, do, and think. Honor your cycles because they all live within you, but be clear that only you can achieve the possibility of navigating the heights. Use the nights you sleep alone as a divine ally that cradles and cares for you in the initiation you have undertaken.

The following rituals will help you activate all this intellectual understanding and manifest it in the experience of sacred sensuality.

☆ RITUAL 22. SACRED SACRUM

1. Lie in bed before sleep and bring your awareness to your pelvic floor. If you are sitting, it is the area that rests on the bed, floor, or chair.
2. Focus on the entire sacral area: the base of the torso where the three pelvic bones fuse and all the muscles that support it, the perineal area, and feel comfortable and soft.
3. On an inhale, squeeze the genital area, as if you want to hold back urine (like *Kegel* exercises).
4. Raise the air up to the spine toward the crown, accompanying this ascending process with a visualization: imagine the air rising through each of the vertebrae in your spine on an upward path.

5. As you exhale, release the tension in the area, leaving the zone relaxed.
6. Repeat this ritual five to seven times while being very aware of your breathing and the pelvic floor closure you are performing. You should also be aware of what happens when you release it.
7. Carefully record your thoughts and emotions before and after this practice. Remember, your breath is what moves the stagnant points so that energy flows freely. You can use a pen and paper to write down what you feel after each practice and keep a conscious journal of your progress. Ask for guidance and messages, especially related to your sensual power and the expansion that will occur as you surrender to lucid dreams.

Purpose and How to Use It

The pelvic floor, an intricate tapestry of muscles and connective tissue, forms the foundation that supports and suspends the pelvic and abdominal organs. Its primary component, the levator ani muscle, spans the pelvic floor, providing a muscular hammock for these vital structures. The pelvic organs can be divided into three compartments: anterior (bladder and urethra), middle (uterus and vagina; prostate and seminal vesicles, in the case of men), and posterior (rectum, anal canal, and sphincter apparatus).

The pelvic floor muscles are primarily supportive structures that help keep the pelvic viscera in place and prevent them from exiting the pelvis when there is tension. This function is achieved through unconscious contraction during rest or conscious contraction during moments of increased intra-abdominal pressure (vomiting, sneezing, coughing, lifting heavy objects, forced expiration). The muscles help maintain both urinary and fecal continence until the appropriate time to evacuate.

Honor the profound significance of this sacred region in the lower part of your body, as it is also home to the perineum (the space between the vagina and the anus), which produces a subtle exchange of energies and vital fluids for your sexual health. When you understand the structure and power of this area, performing this ritual facilitates and clears the path of obstacles to clarify your deepest desires. Embark on this practice before sleep, allowing your entire being to absorb the energetic message: from your sacred area upward, your solitary night becomes a powerful ally in your transformative journey.

In the world of yogis and spiritual seekers, the conscious closure or manipulation of the perineum and sacrum area has great significance, especially when you perform these "closures" at will. In Sanskrit, it is called *mula bandha*. *Mula* means "root or origin" and *bandha* means "closure"; therefore, what occurs is a sealing of the root that is located in the pelvic floor.

Yogis recognize the profound connection between a healthy, supple perineum and balanced mental and emotional clarity regarding sexuality. This translates to the empowered ability to express your desires authentically, saying "no" with confidence and embracing "yes" with enthusiasm. You are the creator and architect of what you choose to live and explore with your sexuality, knowing that in the area of the genitals lies an immense power of spiritual evolution. Likewise, you are the scriptwriter of your own pleasure.

When the root chakra is in balance, you feel vitality, energy, optimism, rejuvenation, and passion that you use throughout the day, as your body recharges from the practice you did at night.

When you perform the sacred sacral ritual and close your mula bandha, you awaken a cascade of benefits. A heightened awareness blooms in this core area of your being. The cerebrospinal fluid surges, forging new pathways for consciousness to flow. You strengthen your identity, which allows you to doubt, change, try, start over, and have great clarity about what you want to do with your sensuality and sexuality. Moreover, the ritual unlocks a deeper understanding of dreams, allowing their messages to illuminate your waking hours.

Document and write about your experiences with this incorporation of root consciousness: the unprecedented doors you will discover will give you a revolutionary perspective on the use and enjoyment of your sexual energy.

☆ RITUAL 23. IMPERIAL CITY

1. Sit on your bed. Lean your back against the pillow so that you are comfortable and feel how the tension leaves your body. Breathe and connect with your heartbeat while bringing your right hand to your throat. Rest it gently so that you can feel it without excessive pressure—just the right touch to acknowledge it.

2. Lower your head so that your chin rests on your hand, between your thumb and index finger. That space in your hands is an exact cavity for you to place your chin comfortably.

3. Focus on your heartbeat as you breathe through your nose, inhaling and exhaling without interfering with the natural flow.

4. Inhale and, when you release the air, contract your glottis by placing your tongue on the back of the palate with your mouth closed. As you contract your glottis, when you exhale, you will hear a sound similar to the wind or ocean waves that comes from your throat (not your nose).

5. While breathing, keep your right hand on your throat and your left hand resting below your navel, at the height of your uterus, the altar of your body.

6. Breathe six or seven times producing the sound and holding your hands on your throat and uterus. When you feel that the circuit is balanced and your mind is serene, begin to massage and caress your body. You can continue breathing in this way or return to your normal breathing.

7. Extend the caress or massage to reach hidden areas—your armpits, between your toes, the insides of your ears—or other places rarely touched.

Purpose and How to Use It

Voluntarily closing the throat and glottis produces an extraordinary energetic reverberation throughout the body and greatly contributes to the development of heightened sensuality. Yogis recommend these closures, or *bandhas* (see the previous perineum closure ritual on page 75), as one of the direct paths to irrigating another consciousness and other levels of understanding. This ritual, by placing your hands on the throat and uterus, connects sacred parts of body areas that are building new genetic information they create, an imperial city with the throat-uterus axis, united by the intelligent center of the heart.

The closed-glottis breathing technique swiftly transmits its vibration to your heart rate, inducing a gentle softening and recalibration. Brain waves slow, ushering you into a meditative state not sleep, but a state of complete, observing presence. In this state, you witness your emotions unfold without identifying with them. In essence, you feel, you allow them expression, yet remain unattached, recognizing them as transient experiences. Throat and perineum, long recognized by mystics for their unique language, resonate together. Your words become a reflection of your womb and cervix, creating a virtuous cycle united by the heart. With this empowered state, victory becomes a natural consequence, not just a visualization.

This entire physical and biological process has a direct correlation with your ability to feel and experience your sexuality, as it triggers the release of hormones and proteins that revitalize you on the deepest level, down to the mitochondria of your cells. Each breath, like ascending a musical octave, refines the tones and frequencies as you recognize that erogenous zones are not societal constructs, but expressions of your inherent sensuality. This energy flows throughout your being, waiting to be discovered.

Wrap yourself in a cocoon of self-awareness each night. Let your throat and mouth become your allies for loving self-talk, whispering words of encouragement and care instead of self-sabotage and despair. Within the sanctuary of your bed, visualize your own imperial city. See it flourish, bathed in light, adorned with vibrant green spaces. This is your haven, ready to welcome you whenever you need it.

☆ RITUAL 24. VIBRATORS AND VIBRATIONS

1. Sitting on the bed, with your back straight and your shoulders away from your ears (to avoid unnecessary tension), take a deep breath, open your mouth, stick out your tongue, and release the breath. Make sure your tongue comes completely out of your mouth so that you can feel more and more space opening up in your throat.
2. Repeat the breathing and activation without fear of the sounds that will come out of your throat. Let them come out freely without holding back and encourage yourself to recognize them as your own. Listen to yourself without judgment or labels; simply let the sounds flow and expand.
3. As you allow your mouth to open wider, visualize a direct connection being created with your vaginal area until you perceive the sound traveling up and down, producing a greater vibration. You will find a more sustained, more constant sound that varies in volume or intensity depending on how you feel.
4. Visualize spaces opening up until you feel your whole body, vibrating and oxygenated, self-generating the transmutation of heavy metals within you into pure gold.
5. Release, and be grateful for the process that occurs with vibration. This high state of appreciation and gratitude is essential for a revealing experience on your magical night carpet.

Purpose and How to Use It

In this ritual, we do not use vibrating devices or insert anything foreign into our bodies. What we do is activate the frequency of these mirror organs, such as the trachea, the vaginal canal, the vocal cords, and the vulva. Practically identical in their anatomy, both ends have this hollow, moist channel, lined with soft tissue, that closes when there is tension and opens when it is relaxed.

The similarities between the throat and the vagina are so striking that if you see drawings or models of both, you cannot tell which is which.

Like inseparable twins who have had their disagreements, they now, finally, become accomplices within you.

Closely touched and connected by the vagus nerve, both organs correspond perfectly with this experience of letting go of the voice, opening the genitals, saying what you feel and think, and expressing what you want. These organs react by closing in the face of threats or tensions and by fully opening with confidence in the face of pleasure and beauty.

As you breathe, sing, eat, move your tongue, and produce sacred saliva, a mirror reflects these acts in your genitals, which receive and feel the same. All this to such an extent that, according to your menstrual cycle, the mucosa and saliva of your throat change, as do the mucosa of the cervix and vaginal acidity.

This ritual invites you to channel the spirits of ancient enchantresses, sorceresses, and wise women, the masters of the spiritual path, the initiators of languages and poems, until the boundaries between your voice and your womb blur. At the level of your cervical vertebrae, your larynx and vocal cords, and the sacred realm of your sacrum, the pelvic region and sexual organs mirror the interconnectedness of all channels and organs. When one suffers, the reflection is imminent in the others. Conversely, when pleasure and love prevail, relaxation cascades throughout your entire being.

Are you ready to awaken sacred sensuality by opening your throat and singing? Singing unlocks a pathway to connect with your sexuality and inner power, independent of external validation. This resonance flows not just upward, but downward as well. The energy you express through your throat can be creative and constructive or dark and draining, just like the vibration emanating from your genital area vagina and cervix, which resonates throughout your entire womb.

This resonance can exist on the biological or spiritual plane, reflecting pleasure or pain, depending on what you decide. You choose what to associate with, but it is essential to understand that everything is interrelated and that, by cultivating well-being in one area, the mirror zone will automatically benefit. Practice the ritual before bed and connect it with the conscious request you make to receive the information you want in your lucid dreams.

☆ RITUAL 25. THE SUNLIGHT BETWEEN YOUR LEGS

1. Find a private place where you can sunbathe, a space where you will not be seen. This could be your patio, a balcony, a corner where the sun comes in through the window and you can be alone.
2. You should do this first thing in the morning or last thing in the afternoon, for a maximum of thirty seconds to one minute.
3. Without underwear, lift your legs so that the sun shines directly on your perineum or choose any position that ensures that the sun reaches your entire genital area.
4. Enjoy everything you feel and record your experience as you do it.
5. At night, in your bed, visualize the light of the great master sun coming out from between your legs. Illuminate your entire kingdom with the energy you charged during the daylight hours.

Purpose and How to Use It

Exposing hidden areas of the body to sunlight is a practice that should be done with common sense but, above all, with clarity of intention. It is a complement to the deep meditations and rituals that you are carrying out with this book and is directly related to the awakening of sensuality in parts of the body that we never, or hardly ever, take into account. A key nerve for the entire pelvic area passes through the perineum, called the pudendal nerve. This nerve and all its complex ramifications make this area more sensitive to sexual sensations and grants awareness of the power you have between your legs. By opening yourself to the sun, you perform a symbolic act of adoration to your genitals in order for them to receive light and heat.

The energy that this modality produces is compared to a high spiritual practice, since it recharges you with vitality and produces a hormonal response that promotes balance and relaxation. Do it once or twice a week for a short period (no more than a minute) and always use the first light of dawn or the last light of the afternoon, so that you do not receive ultraviolet rays that can damage the sensitive skin of the perineum.

The heat and solar energy are gifts that you take to your nocturnal kingdom. You have the power and the right to call on them whenever they are required. Remember again the physical sensation of this warm, gentle sun and visualize how it rises up your spine to the crown of your head, filling tense spaces with relaxation and opening new resonators in your body.

The most beautiful thing about this ritual is that everything that was once hidden can see the light; the world of shadows must be illuminated and the secret parts of your body, those that are taboo or strange to your being, can be revealed to increase your self-perception and elevate your consciousness. At night, you will carry the light of the sun between your legs.

☆ RITUAL 26. THE NOCTURNAL MIRROR OF THE SOUL

1. Find a mirror and take some time to look at your genitals. You can do this in the bathroom before bed or in bed before sleeping. Observe them with consciousness and determination. Let your gaze linger, allowing a connection to form with these intimate areas of your body. Dedicate a few minutes to this practice before drifting off to sleep.

2. As the ritual unfolds, pay close attention to your thoughts and the internal dialogue it evokes. Cultivate a clear intention of letting go of all the opinions that resonate in your head. They are just thoughts: don't get attached to any of them.

3. Look carefully at each of your parts—folds, curves, areas, textures—to identify as many details as possible and familiarize yourself with your splendid body.

4. As you quiet your mind and deepen your observation, bring your awareness to your breath and high-vibrational words. Reframe the reflection in the mirror, naming your genitals with divine, sacred, loving, and elevating terms. Choose words you would use to speak to a cherished loved one, imbuing them

with the same tenderness. Speak to this reflection with the utmost sweetness.

5. Conclude your ritual with a deep appreciation for the discoveries you've made. As you embark on your nocturnal journey, carry this newfound understanding with you, cherishing the miracle of your body as a sacred temple that reflects the essence of your soul in every aspect.

Purpose and How to Use It
Politically incorrect? Culturally inappropriate? Perhaps unfamiliar in some social settings? Have you ever looked at yourself? Do you know your most intimate anatomy? What do you think are the advantages of doing this ritual? Take a mirror and find the most comfortable way to look between your legs at the world that resides there—the world that, in a hidden way, goes with you everywhere. In the mirror you can observe the vulva, encompassing the outer labia majora and the inner labia minora. Notice the clitoris, the perineum, the urethra, the vaginal opening, and the anus.

While you do this, discovering and empowering yourself, you take control of what happens to the erogenous zones of your body; you permit yourself to be part of the whole, even through those regions that are often silenced by cultural constraints. Remember that cultural, political, educational, ancestral, and social mandates restrict free exploration, seeking to keep you submissive and veiled in shame, fueling fear to limit your path to pleasure. This exploration remains shrouded in secrecy, rarely discussed with accurate terms, let alone truly understood; yet, by lifting the veil and activating the practice of looking at yourself, you will encounter your soul, your essence. The ritual of looking at your vulva and other genital areas produces a revolutionary existential movement, just by going down there and observing yourself. It is a calculated and precise meditation that brings the expansive gift of knowing your anatomy, of being curious beyond what anatomy books or posters in the gynecologist's office show you.

You can gaze into your mirror and see the reflection of perfection directly connected to the moon and its cycles, to the mystery of the hidden, to that cosmogony of irrefutable intuition that lies between your legs. Communicate with your feminine genitals, caress them, know them, integrate them, and speak to them sweetly in your nocturnal exploration, before embarking on the spaceship that will take you to the other world, where the stars are your guides.

Guided Meditation for the Mirror

Here is another guided meditation for you to practice while looking in the mirror:

> Observe your face, bringing heightened awareness to each and every detail, allowing thoughts and feelings to arise without judgment. As if performing a sacred ritual, sweep your gaze from your face to your genitals, acknowledging all that makes you whole, like a private communion, a connection activated and cherished by you alone.

The high energy generated by these practices has a phenomenal impact on your daytime experience on a physical, emotional, and mental level. Open yourself up to the synchronicities and miracles that await you.

☆ RITUAL 27. CLITORIS

1. Sit on the bed so that you can feel your sacrum supported by the mattress. Position your body intentionally, with your back straight, avoiding unnecessary tension. Begin abdominal breathing, ensuring that your stomach inflates and deflates to verify that you have transitioned from thoracic breathing and are now using this technique to massage all your internal organs.
2. Engage your perineal closure, or *mula bandha* (as explained in ritual 22 on page 75). Remember to contract the perineal area when you inhale and release it when you exhale. Combine this with diaphragmatic breathing while focusing on the point

between your eyebrows. This serves as a focal point upon which to dedicate your attention to avoid distractions.

3. Now focus on the clitoral area as you move the breath up the spine to the crown of the head. Each inhalation starts from the clitoris and moves up. In the meantime, choose whether you will use your hands to touch yourself or continue with the breathing practice only (if you choose this, I want you to know that you will be entering a much more advanced technique of self-knowledge, feel free to try it and explore).

4. Feel and visualize a radiance that covers you, activated by your breathing. This will give you an intimate and novel relationship with what is going on inside you. You can use the practice to ask for the specific things you want, desire, or need. You can even go into particular matters, such as healing health issues, resolving conflicts, opening opportunities, and so on, while keeping the vision and the point between your eyebrows.

5. Practice this nightly ceremony before bed. Take advantage of the new hormonal levels you will produce with the ritual, as they will balance any disruption in your flow of energy. It is a practice of high mystical value that also activates visions and opens a channel to receive messages from more evolved entities. These invisible benefactors enhance your frequency, your self-love and your trust in your path.

Purpose and How to Use It

Forgotten, buried, unnamed, repudiated for centuries of machismo and human misconceptions, denied by scientists and doctors, the clitoris, your clitoris, wants to speak, to be heard, to have prominence and space in your existence, to be reborn thanks to your will and decision. Its name comes from the Greek *kleitoris* and translates to "small hill," an etymology that already belittles and diminishes it, although its power is undeniable and its absolute belonging to the feminine makes it invincible.

The clitoris is the only organ in the human body that exists solely for pleasure. Boasting over eight thousand nerve endings (double that of the penis), it's a masterpiece of blood vessels, glands, and intricate structures understood intimately by women. Both the clitoris and the penis share a common origin, developing from the same embryonic tissue. At eight weeks of gestation, however, the Y chromosome in male DNA triggers the transformation of this tissue into a penis, while in females, it becomes the magnificent clitoris. This female-exclusive organ is made up of three parts: the *glans*, the visible tip veiled by the labia minora, mirroring the male foreskin; the *body*, comprised of two corpora cavernosa structures; and the *roots*, anchoring it firmly to the pubic bone.

It is essential to know and understand its anatomy, because the fact that it is hidden inside the pelvis gives it mysterious capabilities. Thus, it is crucial that you take ownership of what belongs to you and fully control this organ of pleasure. This ritual teaches you and invites you to explore your clitoris with the full awareness that the energy that you generate in these encounters with yourself is a source of health and vitality that you must take care of and preserve.

With each conscious breath taken while focusing on your third eye, you ignite a cascade of spiritual awakening. This sacred act elevates the experience to your third eye chakra, facilitating the decalcification of your pineal and pituitary glands. It gently encourages the loving flow of cerebrospinal fluid, transforming the luminous sparks you generate within into a potent reservoir for restoring balance to your body, mind, and emotions. By doing that you cast aside any lingering shame or societal impositions, inherited from a bygone era. Embrace this ritual to bathe yourself in light before embarking on your nightly dreams, soaring through the celestial realm of your magnificent night time.

☆ RITUAL 28. EROTICISM EVERYWHERE

1. You can choose to sit or lie down on your bed. Before drifting off to sleep, gently massage the back of your ears, moving upward and downward. Notice the cartilage, its shape and

texture, as if you're experiencing it for the first time. Close your eyes to heighten the physical sensation and use both hands simultaneously to create a rhythmic motion while breathing slowly.

2. Now, move on to your earlobes and the surrounding tissues, continuing the massage with the same rhythm and intensity. Keep your eyes closed; if thoughts arise, let them pass without judgment. As you touch your ears, place your index fingers inside them and gently press down for a few moments, calming your nervous system and activating the vagus nerve. Afterward, simply pay attention to what you feel.

3. With the same intensity, continue downward, touching your neck and nape as if it's the first time you've done so. What do you feel there? Anything new? Did any emotional shifts occur when you reached this area?

4. Now, use your fingers to stretch your forehead three times, moving from the center outward. Next, move to your eyebrows, performing a circular massage from the center toward the temples. Then, go from the under-eye area to the cheeks. Linger there, feeling the cheekbones (bones, skin, textures), and move on to your lips, gently touching them while honoring the memories and emotions they may evoke. Take this step of the ritual to celebrate your eroticism and sensuality.

5. Now that you've completed the journey across your face, continue breathing softly. Remember that this contact activates every cell in your body. You can repeat the circuit several times until you fall asleep. Breathe: in the world of dreams, truths about the infinite power of your eroticism as a driving force in life will be revealed to you.

Purpose and How to Use It

Beyond the known erotic zones, such as the clitoris or nipples, the face, head, and neck of women have an explosive power when it comes to communicating pleasure. This ritual invites you on a voyage of discovery that you should embark on without prejudice or expectation as you begin the dynamic exploration of these areas of your body. Your lips, for example, have more than a million nerve endings, making them one of the most exposed erogenous zones of the body. The slightest touch, contact, or rub sends a cascade of information to your brain, activating neurotransmitters and hormones that influence how you think and feel.

Watch what happens within you as you do the ritual, as you bring together all these parts of high erotic power that are fully interconnected and that, when turned on during the night, will put your body in a state of grace. These areas, in addition to their connection with your eroticism, touch all points related to your vagus nerve—fundamental in calming the sympathetic nervous system and releasing tensions and irritations. When you perform this massage, your parasympathetic system, the system of calm and patience, is activated and renewed, bringing countless benefits to your brain, emotions, and physical body.

In addition to their impact on your body, the areas you touch during this massage are directly related to your lymphatic system, which is responsible for draining toxins, waste products, pathogens, dead blood cells, impurities, and everything your body doesn't need through a network of tissues and organs. It is mainly composed of lymph, a fluid that contains white blood cells that defend the body against germs, and lymphatic vessels, which transport lymph throughout the body. The primary organs of the lymphatic system are the thymus and bone marrow.

This magnificent system does not have a pump to propel fluids (like the circulatory system); therefore, lymph flows thanks to the movements of the body, the pulsation of the arteries, and the contractions of the muscles. Lymph is a colorless liquid containing white blood cells, hence its poetic name, which comes from the Latin *lympha*, "clear water," moving throughout the body and keeping fluid levels balanced in order to prevent infections and abrupt health failures.

For its cleansing mission to work, the body must be in motion. What is not activated stagnates. When paralyzed by the head's negativity, the body succumbs to a drama of catastrophic narratives; therefore, this sensual and intimate ritual seeks to connect you with nontraditional erogenous parts of the body and, in doing so, allows you to understand that you are contributing to the overall well-being of your organism, accompanying the lymph in its cleansing dance throughout your body.

As you cultivate this awakened eroticism, a crescendo of self-discovery unfolds. Through this practice, questions about your being and the power held within your body will inevitably arise. These questions are yours alone to answer. Do the ritual in your solitary bed and let your imagination fly without limits or fear, because nothing and no one will interrupt it. After you have finished, initiate a dialogue with the back of your ears, earlobes, neck, forehead, eyebrows, eyes, cheeks, and lips. Ask them how they feel now that you are pampering them. Ask them and listen carefully to the response of each one of them, because what they tell you will result in a widening of your field of vision and feelings.

Embark on a transformative journey of consciousness expansion, as your hands become conduits of divine touch, awakening unconventional erogenous zones to a symphony of sensations.

CHAPTER FIVE

LUCID DREAMING

Women, immerse yourselves in this poem by Borges. Savor each of his words, as they will be the prelude to your lucid dreaming journey. Feel his verses course through your being, making them your own. His words weave a tapestry of dreams' complexity, while at the same time revealing their inherent simplicity as a wellspring of guidance for your waking life. Universal literature and great poets and writers have spoken countless times about the world of dreams; the mystery that inhabits their territories and the questions that arise between the worlds of sleep and wakefulness.

Do you ever awaken with a dream clinging stubbornly to your mind, its images and sensations lingering for days or even weeks? Perhaps you've encountered situations or people within these dreams, individuals whom you do not recognize from your waking life. What stirs within you when a dream's vivid information feels like a premonition, leaving you unsure of its meaning or how to act upon it? In my experience, whenever I dream about certain people, I always wonder if they have also dreamed about me. I wonder if we have met in that dreamlike, surreal, indecipherable, timeless, and illogical realm for a reason I don't understand.

In this poem, Borges plunges into the existential abyss of dreams, grappling with the enigma of the dreamer and the dreamed, creator and creation. He confronts the profound question: are we mere figments in a deity's dream, or is our so-called wakefulness simply a continuation of the grand narrative spun by a cosmic dreamer? Breathe deeply, and let the poem wash over you, its mysteries slowly unraveling.

> *Why is it so sad to be awake at dawn?*
> *It strips us of a gift so strange, so deep,*
> *It can be remembered only in half-sleep,*
> *Moments of drowsiness that gild and adorn*
> *The waking mind with dreams...*
>
> JORGE LUIS BORGES,
> TRANSLATED BY ROBERT MEZEY

In the captivating prologue of his magnificent book, *The Tibetan Yogas of Dream and Sleep*, Tibetan teacher Tenzin Wangyal Rinpoche states: "We spend a third of our lives asleep. No matter what we do, whether our activities are virtuous or not, whether we are saints or murderers, monks or libertines, every day ends the same way. We close our eyes and dissolve into darkness. We do this without fear, even though everything we know as 'self' disappears."

Thus, we embark on these out-of-body journeys, astrally limitless, filled with stories that appear in the form of images—some so tangible that we are literally "awake" in sleep; others blurred, but always intriguing. That is why this book invites you time and time again to dare to do something transcendental, to evolve your whole being by establishing an initiatory path as a priestess of your dreams.

In this chapter, I'll share with you a wealth of information, practical experiences, and concrete data to help you embark on a magical journey that will awaken a new consciousness within your entire being. You will witness clear and tangible physical, mental, and emotional changes, especially in your relationships with yourself and others, and in your perception of the world. You will also feel an unwavering confidence in your ability to navigate mental noise and chaos and put an end to patterns of suffering and ancestral burdens.

☆ RITUAL 29. MNEMONIC TECHNIQUE

1. Before you drift off to sleep and enter deep slumber, relax in your bed. Now, focus your attention on a recent dream you remember and bring it fresh to your memory with the intention of picking up where you left off. If you have it written down, review the notes as they will be an aid in bringing that specific moment to mind just before sleep, leading to the production of a lucid dream.

2. It is essential that in this recollection of a recent dream you clearly identify a dream element, something surreal that makes it clear in your mind that it is a dream—what is called a *dreamsign*. If you remember, for example, a dream from the previous night, focus your attention on something bizarre that could only happen in the dream world and would not happen in the waking state. Like flying, talking to people who have died, seeing people turn into animals, or vice versa.

3. Remember the dream. Focus on the dreamsign and hold it in your memory. Before sleep, repeat three times aloud, "I will remember that I am dreaming, I will remember that I am dreaming, I will remember that I am dreaming."

4. Visualize yourself transforming the memory of your dream into a lucid dream. In other words, imagine that you consciously know that you are in the dream, that you are both the dream and the dreamer.

5. Now that you are done with your practice, close your eyes and surrender to sleep. Do so with confidence that you will have the experience you desire.

Purpose and How to Use It

Mnemonics, a memory-hacking technique commonly used for exams and tests, empowers you to remember what you wish. In this case, you will use the resource to connect with your ability to consciously produce a lucid dream and begin to explore the information it delivers. By repeating, as you fall asleep, that when you dream you will know you are dreaming, you start an induction of your memory into the lucidity of what you will experience during the night. Just as the step-by-step ritual indicates, you must be precise in identifying that you are in a dream, using some element that could only happen in that state—unreal situations, indescribable places, encounters with beings that are not there or otherworldly things, among others.

Once you have registered the dream and its dreamlike characteristic, you activate the intention to continue with that plot. In the middle of the situation, you "wake up without waking up"; in this way, you will be aware that you are dreaming. When you achieve this, you can ask, inquire, talk to the protagonists who have information and messages for you, change things, and use the dream as an oracle of what you want to achieve.

Patience and self-compassion are essential during this practice, as it may take several months to achieve lucid dreaming. However, depending on your emotional and physical state, it could happen much sooner. The key is to approach this realm with a high degree of curiosity and minimal fear, so that you can fully explore the path it offers. Approach it with great inquisitiveness to see what happens, what emerges, and what you understand.

☆ RITUAL 30. CLEAR THE RIGHT NOSTRIL

1. Lie down with your head on the pillow, resting on the left side to clear the right nostril.
2. While your left nostril touches the pillow, place your left hand on your cheek, applying gentle pressure to your head, ensuring that the left nostril remains covered.
3. Bend your legs in a fetal position so that your body is balanced. Rest on your left hip as you feel relaxed and continue breathing smoothly, with total tranquility (no sound of inhalation and exhalation).
4. Focus your attention on the throat (communication chakra)

and imagine or visualize an open and fragrant lotus flower in this part of your body, inhabiting your vocal cords and neck.
5. With this body position, start to relax and feel your heartbeat. Repeat the phrase: "I will remember that I am dreaming," until you feel that you are starting to fall into a deep sleep.

Purpose and How to Use It
Originating from Tibetan Buddhism, this practice is known as dream yoga. It employs a combination of postures, breathing techniques, and visualizations to activate profound states of consciousness, transitioning from the body to the mind, as a form of nocturnal meditation during sleep. It fosters observation and familiarity with the nature of your mind, encompassing the vastness of possibilities within the visions produced by your body, unfolding in a progression as follows: you learn to recall your dreams, then become adept at awakening within your dreams, subsequently, you train your mind during the dream state, and ultimately translate this into your waking life with an elevated level of consciousness beyond the ordinary.

To comprehend this specific ritual and its deep spiritual meaning it is important to understand that, for Tibetan Buddhism, there is an energetic channel in each nostril that relates to the cerebral hemispheres and is divided according to gender. In the case of women, the left nostril is white and connects with deeper and more intimate emotions; the right nostril is red and connects with expansive wisdom energies while the central channel is blue and balances both parts. For the Buddhist system of dream yoga, the channels are reversed according to your gender; therefore, in the case of men, the white one is related to expansive wisdom and the red one to intimacy, which explains why we women are instructed to sleep on our left side and men on their right side.

Both nostrils must function properly to generate balancing hormones and positive emotional states, and in order to become facilitators for some aspects of spiritual evolution. Depending on how we breathe—the nostril that is more active, the way we let air enter and leave the body—we will achieve understanding and evolution in both the dream and waking world.

In the Tibetan Buddhist practice of dream yoga, for women, the left nostril is the one that moves more negativity; therefore, it is recommended that it be placed on the pillow during the night, allowing the right red channel to take center stage in cleansing the physical, emotional, and mental bodies, while the blue or central channel, that of nonduality, brings the opposites to a middle point of calm and unity.

The ritual emphasizes sleeping on your left side for a crucial reason. Your prana, or vital life force, needs unimpeded flow—guided by your breath—to ensure your rest forms a clean and perfect canvas for your daily aspirations. While dreaming, your brain actively generates a world of images and movement, and this very activity nourishes your breath. This dynamic interplay between prana and breath is why posture and breathing technique are essential for achieving lucid dreams. Sleep loses its static quality when fueled by the force of prana.

Perform this ritual at least once a week. This will allow your body and unconscious mind to become accustomed to properly cleansing your channels and will facilitate your quest for lucid dreams. Your body's cells are conductors of electricity: they collect, transmit, and store energy that expands throughout your body. As they pass through your bones with their iron deposits, they produce high levels of magnetism, making you the mothership that connects the ether with Mother Earth.

Enjoy the process deeply as you find your posture and surrender to the pleasure of flying alone!

☆ RITUAL 31. NINE ROUND*

1. Sit on your bed with your back straight, being very mindful to avoid creating unnecessary tension in your spine (hands relaxed, shoulders away from your ears, arms slightly separated from your body). Breathe in and out through your nose. Remember

---

*A version of ritual 50 from my book *Enciende tu corazón* (Ignite Your Heart).

to keep your mouth relaxed and your tongue touching the area of the palate where your front teeth begin. Take two or three conscious breaths and begin your practice.

2. Cover the left nostril with the index finger of your right hand and inhale through the right.
3. Now cover the right nostril and exhale through the left, imagining that all the accumulated anger and rage are leaving your body.
4. Repeat two more times, clearly visualizing the cleansing you are carrying out. You no longer have anger, rage, resentment, or irritation in your system.
5. Now do it in reverse: cover the right nostril and inhale through the left.
6. Cover the left and release through the right while visualizing all of your attachments coming out: greed, gluttony, and avarice.
7. Repeat two more times. With each exhale, list everything you suffer when you attach yourself to things and people, situations and memories, to the desire to keep and possess excessively instead of letting go and detaching.
8. Now, inhale through both nostrils and, as you exhale, imagine releasing all ignorance and confusion from your mind. Imagine that your ideas are becoming clearer, that you listen to the intelligence of your heart to make decisions, and that you become clear—crystal clear—about your present and future.
9. Repeat this twice, while inhaling and exhaling: "I am ready to let go of what I don't need; I am ready to be reborn in every moment. In my lucid dream I will find what I am looking for. I breathe and surrender to my nightly spiritual retreat."

Purpose and How to Use It
This breathwork ritual acts as a powerful equalizer, balancing emotions and purging what no longer serves you, both mentally and physically. It cleanses the body's subtle energy channels, allowing you to release

negativity such as selfishness, anger, and attachment. With each exhale, you consciously shed feelings of greed, lack of compassion, and confusion. This process leads to a profound self-rediscovery, free from shame or judgment. Within the sanctuary of your bed, poised for lucid dreaming, you experience a complete renewal of body and spirit.

The emotions that this ritual cleanses are very fast and clever, they blend seamlessly with sadness or euphoria and are so deeply rooted in your existence that they will fight to the last breath to remain a part of your life.

As you do this ritual, you will clearly feel the resistance of anger, the willpower of greed, and the hold of ignorance and confusion. However, you are ready and you know what to do to make these frequencies fade away in order to make room for new things, fresh ideas, and abstract concepts that before seemed unattainable. In the ritual of these nine rounds, you will conquer them.

The beauty of this ritual lies in its flexibility; you can perform it at any point during your evening preparation. With a bit of practice, you'll even be able to discern the air entering and exiting the desired nostril without covering it, perceiving the red and the white, and the blue of unity within the central channel.

This practice creates space for egotistical perspectives to dissipate and altruistic thoughts to flourish. It allows you to release what no longer serves you, making room for the construction of lucid dreams, which, without inner cleansing, take much longer to manifest.

It's an excellent strategy for detachment without drama. It's the true "letting go" that brings no complaints or victimization, but rather a sense of profound and complete freedom. You'll feel as though you've given yourself a thorough internal cleansing, removing stagnant and entrenched elements, situations, and emotions that were swept under the rug. You allow the unconscious, the vast intelligence that lies beneath the surface, to flow freely, leading you into the vast world of dreams, cleansed and pristine. Just as you bathe before bed, this is your inner shower.

☆ RITUAL 32. WAKE UP EARLY

1. Hop into your magic bed and set your alarm to go off approximately two hours before your usual waking time. For example, if you typically wake up at 7:00 am, set your alarm for 5:00 am.
2. Upon waking, take a few deep breaths and sit up in bed with the intention of having a lucid dream experience as impeccably as possible. Sitting up helps you achieve a higher quality state of wakefulness. Remain seated for one or two minutes.
3. At this point, consciously activate your intention to wake up within your dreams, taking advantage of the early morning hours. Make sure you repeat: "I will remember that I am dreaming."
4. Before falling back asleep, remember to reset your alarm to your usual waking time. Lie back down on your left side, keeping your right nostril clear.
5. Return to sleep after this intentional interruption. Upon waking, write down everything you can recall from your dreams.

Purpose and How to Use It

Lucid dreams consistently occur during the REM stage, also known as paradoxical sleep, when the brain is active and the muscles are relaxed (see Stages of Sleep on page 14). Each of the five stages of sleep directly correlates with brain activity, even more dynamically than in our waking state. This intricate dance between brain waves holds the key to unlocking the dream world.

Beta and Alpha waves are associated with being awake, while Theta and Delta arise in the moment of sleep. In the transition of brain waves from Beta to Alpha, a presleep state called *hypnagogia* occurs when you start to fall asleep but are still aware that you are passing into another state, an intermediate state that we commonly call *half-sleep*. This moment can sometimes resemble what happens during deep meditation, when we lose the boundary between being asleep and awake and enter unexplored spaces, flowing between the conscious and the unconscious. Remember that the first stage of sleep lasts between five and ten minutes, when Alpha brain waves decrease to Theta and move into the second stage, when we enter a slightly deeper sleep, slower breath, as well as heart rate and body temperature.

As we enter stages three and four, our brain waves slow down to Delta—a state of deep sleep where the body is restored, tissues are repaired, growth hormone is produced, and healing occurs at the cellular level. For about thirty minutes, the body and brain remain in this stage before entering REM sleep (you may experience the sensation of stage two, half-sleep, before entering REM sleep), as the brain returns to a high level of activity, almost with the same daytime frequencies. At this time, breathing and heartbeat accelerate while the muscles are completely paralyzed. This state is so impactful that your body consumes more oxygen in REM sleep than when you are awake, in a cycle that repeats four to five times a night, in periods of ninety minutes.

During these cycles, there are moments (up to fifteen times a night) when you wake up without being aware of it; this is when you move, change position, kick. All sleep research confirms that the REM state is not reached in the first part of the night, but rather in the second part; so, waking up voluntarily two hours earlier than usual prepares the brain for a higher quality and quantity of lucid dreams.

Therefore, it is about an hour before waking up that REM periods intensify; this is known as dream primetime. The recommendation is to perform this ritual as indicated: take advantage of the first hours of sleep to recover and rest, and use the last hours for the magic of lucid dreaming. The more familiar you become with this dynamic and routine, the stronger the messages, answers, and signals you will receive through your dreams.

☆ RITUAL 33. LUCID MEDITATORS

1. Sit on your bed. Choose a space in the middle, on the central meridian, so that you receive, in a balanced way, the energy that comes from the East and the West. Breathe. Bring the fingers of

both hands to your forehead and, resting your fingertips, gently produce the sound "aum," while visualizing the color violet covering your entire head. Feel the vibration that is generated from your forehead throughout your body and stretch the pronunciation of the letter "m" at the end: "aummmmmmmmmmm."

2. Now, move on to the throat area and, with your fingers resting there, produce the sound "ha." Visualize the color blue covering your entire neck and nape. The vibration that is created here can be felt throughout your back side, including the backs of your legs.

3. Use both hands to reach your heart, producing the sound "hum" and visualize the area and everything around it in green. This is your heart center charged with emotional intelligence; therefore, while doing this part of the ritual, visualize your heart expanding and growing.

4. Once you are familiar with the three sounds, do it as a harmonic repetition that resonates throughout your entire body. Do seven rounds before lying down in your bed on your left side so that the right nostril is clear and you can enter the deepest sleep state, with these three frequencies vibrating through the mitochondria of your cells.

Purpose and How to Use It

Lucid meditation focuses on balancing three fundamental points. These points achieve a basic equilibrium when producing high-frequency dreams. Remember that the states of sleep and wakefulness are entirely interdependent; therefore, if you improve the quality of what happens during the night, your day will inevitably change for the better.

In the first step of this ritual, using the sound "aum" and the color violet while touching your forehead, melts mental icebergs, or a stagnation of ideas that seem impossible to break. By producing this sound and connecting its associated color, you will begin to befriend your power to destroy the rigid and square structures that only impede your evolution; it is as simple as touching your forehead, the place of the prefrontal cortex that activates discernment, good reasoning, and the ability to make nonviolent choices.

In the second step of the ritual, as you repeat "ha" deep in your throat, associating the sound to an intense blue color, you feel the vibration of your vocal cords and the lubrication it generates for your voice and words, opening you up to a new kind of communication, free from rules and learned structures. Your beautiful words—agile, vital, compassionate toward yourself and others—and the poetry of your verbs—molding your existence, opening you to true transmutation and alchemy—will finally lead you to the zone of your heart, where you say "hum."

This is the heart center, beating with determination and rejuvenation to the rhythm of the sound with its associated green color. Here you are breaking down prejudices, opening to love and compassion, and expanding the heart's electromagnetic field to reach beyond, in support of a new narrative that encompasses the frequency of encountering yourself in all dimensions, from the territory of your bed to the universe.

These three points correspond with your mind, your speech, and your body, so it is your duty and obligation to keep them vibrant and vital. Notice how the information from your lucid dreams flows much better when you achieve coherence between these three parts.

If you work with lucidity, observing your mind during the day, this focus will be transferred and translated into your nocturnal dreams. Everything is interconnected. By consciously collaborating your daytime and nighttime experiences, you can profoundly support yourself in your healing and growth processes. For the Buddhist practice of dream yoga, lucid dreams have a spiritual and consciousness-raising purpose—to the point that some masters proclaim that a single lucid dream is worth much more than all of the spiritual practice done during the day.

☆ RITUAL 34. THE THREE R'S OF LUCID DREAMING

This is a ritual to perform upon waking up.

- **Rewrite**: Immediately upon waking, write down whatever you remember of your dream. Try to do this as quickly as possible so that the images don't slip away. Create a narrative or sequence in which you include and acknowledge the *dreamsign* (see ritual 29 on page 93)—the unusual or illogical elements that only appear in dreams.
- **Rehearse**: Imagine that you are back in the dream, but this time the new version of you is lucid. Repeat the visualization as if you were rehearsing a role in a play, and do it as many times as you need until you see yourself clearly back in the dream—what was happening, the setting around you, whether or not there were people, and so on.
- **Recall**: Create a mental reminder during the day so that when you go back to bed and begin the process of entering your lucid dream, you know that you are dreaming and continue to be fully aware of the dreamsign you chose when you rewrote and rehearsed it.

Purpose and How to Use It

By activating the Three R ritual, you will unlock a heightened state of perception, sharpening your peripheral vision and fostering a conscious connection between your heart and brain. As you delve into the realm of sleep, you will encounter dreamsigns, vivid events that hold a high probability of mirroring reality while you rest. To connect with these dreamsigns, consistent practice and a heightened awareness of their potential occurrence are essential.

Upon waking, meticulously record your dreams, underlining elements that stand out as particularly specific and indicative of a dream state. Compile these elements into a list, serving as a reference point for recognizing dreamsigns during subsequent deep sleep episodes. Implement concrete intention-setting strategies to decisively establish your awareness within the dream, enabling you to maintain a state of participatory lucidity.

Remember, dreamsigns serve as beacons, illuminating your consciousness within the dream realm while simultaneously activating an altered perception when you are awake. The world around you will transform, transcending the confines of three-dimensional perception into a territory of boundless expansion and coherence.

In this ritual, I ask you to be extremely aware of the universes that will begin to appear before you and, above all, of the amount of information you will receive from the universal source directly in your inner being. As this ritual connects the transition from night to day, it is important to include a morning practice of mental hygiene before you start your daily routines. Meditate every day to have absolute clarity about what you want and what you wish to receive.

☆ RITUAL 35. THE PALACE OF FLEXIBILITY

1. Engage in some light yoga, stretches, or poses that activate your spine and can be done naturally in bed. These include bringing your legs to one side or the other, raising them and placing them against the headboard or wall, stretching your arms, and opening and closing your hands quickly.

2. You can also perform the cat-cow yoga pose, getting on all fours and moving your spine up and down. Raise your head by curving your back inward; then bring your head to your chin by curving your back upward, just like a bristling cat. It is also recommended to make circular movements while sitting on the bed, with your legs crossed and your hands on your knees, making sure that your chest expands when you go forward and bringing your chin to your chest when you go backward. All these stretches open areas that concentrate a lot of trauma and pain and help release them.

3. As you stretch, recall the characteristic elements of your dreamsigns and, if necessary, review your dream notes from previous

days. This starts to occupy your brain with imagery conducive to accessing your dreams without obstacles when you go to sleep.

4. Focus on the channel in your spine. Imagine your vertebrae are like flexible gold coins stacked on top of each other. This treasure activates new neural networks and opens luminous paths for ideas to flow and grow in your mind while you are aware of moving energy, life, and cerebrospinal fluid. This is the promoter of rejuvenation and vital presence that fills your palace of flexibility with grace and abundance.

5. Once your spine is relaxed and supple, lie down and begin your process of entering sleep. Do so with confidence and tranquility, knowing that your sacred spaces are lubricated and activated, and that your systems are in perfect balance.

Purpose and How to Use It

Your spine is miraculous—a silent pillar of support. It allows you to move and feel, sending cerebrospinal fluid that flows effortlessly through it, protecting your brain and spinal cord. This substance, rich in glucose, vitamins, hormones, amino acids, nucleic acids, electrolytes, and white blood cells, ensures that the entire central nervous system is always well-oxygenated and nourished. It deserves to be known and honored by you, as it plays an essential role in your lucid dreaming process and, above all, in the power you gain when you become familiar with it as a tool while you are sleeping alone.

The movement of your spine creates a smooth highway for the various functions of this fluid: nourishing the central nervous system, carrying oxygen and nutrients to the cells of the brain and spinal cord, maintaining internal pressure so that the brain and spinal cord do not suffer. It plays a crucial role in homeostasis, acting as a shock absorber, protecting the brain from its own weight. The cerebrospinal fluid also boasts a robust immune system, safeguarding against infections, and acting as a courier—transporting essential hormones that keep the entire neurological network functioning flawlessly.

Embrace the marvels of your body to cultivate lucid dreams. The most proactive approach lies in gaining a deeper understanding of your organism's inner workings. Equipped with adequate bodily information, your brain will respond in accordance with your intentions. Conscious awareness of your spine and its remarkable adaptability will inevitably translate into more meaningful, productive dreams, brimming with insights and answers to your pressing questions.

The clear instruction is to consciously envision creating a palace of flexibility, akin to constructing your dream house. Meticulously incorporate every detail and object that resonates with you and adorn it with colors and decor that stir your heart, knowing that the palace's upkeep rests entirely upon your shoulders.

Activate your spine, allowing perspective and intuition to flow seamlessly through each vertebra, and surrender to sleep with unwavering confidence and radiance in order to witness the unfolding of this miraculous experience.

CHAPTER SIX

AWAKEN THE HEART OF THE WORLD

Imagine the power of your heart's brain when you sleep alone: when there are no sensory disturbances of any kind and you can play, delve, explore, and blatantly be curious to achieve everything you want. No longer is there time to pretend or feel shy; rather, it is time to show yourself limitlessly in your emotional and physical exploration. You are already a walking manifesto, a woman who flows and sees things with a sharp mind and an enchanted heart. Emotions send signals from the center of the chest to the heart's electromagnetic field—a field that expands up to six times more than that of the brain and acquires extreme lucidity at night.

The melatonin that is produced from your pineal gland, in perfect quantity, balances with your heartbeat and brain waves. When you are alone and not sharing a bed, the expansion and superior understanding that you acquire physically and emotionally opens up.

Your heartbeat is a channel that sends messages to each of your cells. You can program this channel with elevated feelings such as love, compassion, gratitude, and appreciation. In this way, you regulate the activity of the sympathetic nervous system and increase the activity of the parasympathetic nervous system (the sympathetic is your accelerator and the parasympathetic is your brake).

Remember, your heart is not a metronome, but quite the opposite. Its rhythm and variability (heart rate variability) change according to what you feel, think, and how you breathe.

Variability exists even when you sleep and is regulated by the autonomic nervous system; therefore, if this system is not balanced, your heart beats irregularly, your brain waves are altered, and your emotions are overflowing. How you breathe and what you think and feel promote chaos or coherence, confusion or fusion. Your lucid dreams and the power of your nocturnal sensuality create algorithms that can favor either tremendous success or mediocre living; these options are always available, at your fingertips, and no one can take them away from you. You choose. You decide; you are responsible for your life, sculpting the work of art that you want to be.

You have the power to modify your biology, to change your genetic information, to produce new neural connections by filling your cells with conscious nutrition and providing a new environment for each of them. Break free from statements and agreements that force you to "inherit diseases" and condemn you to repeat stories of drama and suffering.

Observe the ebb and flow of ideas and thoughts, letting them pass as if you were watching a loose cloud in the sky. This is the beginning of the journey of self-knowledge and self-regulation. You can give this gift to yourself as you begin to love from the heartbeat of your full and overflowing heart, unveiling the new being you will come to recognize during the solitary and divine night.

BEATING IN COHERENCE

How beautiful it is when you perceive your life, actions, words, and thoughts in a coherent way. Here, the marvelous clarity of ideas takes place, the certainty filled with faith and consistently synchronized in all your aspects.

In the field of heart coherence, this translates into a state of balance between the mind, heart, emotions, and physical body, which intertwine, cocreating in community with your peers, family, and the world around you. A social coherence is perceived as a stable group with aligned relationships, in which you use your energy to optimize collective cohesion. Likewise, it harmonizes your emotions and deepest desires with a conviction of high individual freedom and group responsibility.

Where you focus your attention is where you put your energy; where you apply your will and discipline, you can manifest all that you desire. To achieve this, it is essential to shift your focus to your body, prioritizing your heart center, and to practice self-hypnosis in a calm and positive state. Set your intention very clearly, breathing from the center of your chest, until each inhalation and exhalation is rhythmic and accompanied by high-frequency emotions. This immediately produces a cardiac coherence effect that balances your brain, allowing different regions to operate in harmony and achieve optimal levels of communication and coordination in both hemispheres.

Surrender to the night, to flying on the magic carpet of your bed from the deep coherence of all your visible and invisible bodies, while inviting the unknown to be a part of your journey. Enjoy and revel in it!

☆ RITUAL 36. NOCTURNAL HEART

1. Lie down in bed and feel your body completely relax. Surrender to the support of the mattress, begin to breathe from the center of your chest, locating the inhalation and exhalation there. Imagine and visualize the air entering and leaving from that area in the middle of your body and, consciously, make it slower and deeper than normal.

2. Produce an intentional regulation of breathing at a rate of ten seconds (inhale for five seconds and exhale for five seconds), creating the heart-coherence frequency while keeping your eyes closed and feeling a state of deep and complete calm.

3. To experience the coherence, do the mental counting in this way: when you inhale, count to five and when you exhale, do the

same. Remember, your abdominal or diaphragmatic breathing will help you in concentration and mindfulness.

4. Repeat the sequence for a couple of minutes, while you fall asleep, so that your heart's brain is properly active during the night. You will produce an electromagnetic field connected to the Earth's heartbeat and your nocturnal journey will be a portal for your spiritual and emotional growth.

Purpose and How to Use It

As you drift into the night, within your spaceship of dreams, your heart slows its rhythm, the nervous system quiets its hum, and much of your body's activity slows down too. Within five minutes of entering the realm of light sleep, your heartbeat enters a restful state, typically dropping to around sixty beats per minute, while the symphony of your nervous system undergoes a gentle shift.

Not only does the heart rate slow down, but body temperature drops, muscles relax, and, in deep sleep, blood pressure drops and your heart rate slows down between 20 percent and 30 percent below resting heart rate.

During REM sleep, your dreams become a captivating reality show, with your heart rate mirroring the action. Imagine a scenario where you're running in your dream—your heart races just as it would during a waking jog. Therefore, the brain in the center of your chest should be acknowledged and used to your advantage during sleep, as your personal trainer in the art of diving into your unconscious.

As you sleep alone during your spiritual retreat, sinking into the mattress, the nightly heart ritual unfolds a spectrum of possibilities for your body and mind but, above all, for your spiritual development and evolution.

This practice aims to foster a deep nighttime coherence between the brain of your heart and the one in your skull so that the productivity you obtain from those hours of sleep will be high-performance for your waking moments as well. You can take advantage of your spiritual retreat to program your heart's desires and needs and to seek greater understanding or answers to your questions. In this way, you will wake up with clear and lucid ideas about what you need to do and the direction to take with your decisions.

☆ RITUAL 37. BRIGHT MIND, KIND HEART

1. Settle into a comfortable seated position on your bed before drifting off to sleep. Begin by scanning your body from head to toe, consciously releasing any tension, particularly in your feet and hands. Focus your attention on the area of your heart, noticing its rhythm and beat, allowing yourself to be carried by its melody.
2. Envision your breath emanating from this central point within your chest. You may bring your hands together in a prayer-like position, the gentle touch serving as a reminder to return to a state of mindful presence as you connect with your heartbeat.
3. Cultivate a regenerative sentiment within this area, such as compassion, understanding, kindness, gratitude, or love. Be clear in your choice, as each emotion carries a distinct vibrational frequency. Select one and remain focused, avoiding distractions.
4. Intentionally visualize the radiation of this revitalizing feeling toward others. Encompass those closest to you, acquaintances, and even those who pose challenges in your life—your "enemies" or those with whom you hold unresolved debts, whether emotional or physical. Include everyone in your emanation of elevated consciousness.
5. If your mind wanders, gently return your attention to your breathing. Employ a five-second count for both inhalation and exhalation to effectively refocus your attention.

This technique supports you in creating new patterns and maintaining the coherence of your cranial brain and heart brain for longer periods. It is excellent to do before bed, because the transformation begins in your unconscious mind and moves to your conscious mind, bringing about fundamental changes in your entire being.

Purpose and How to Use It

On your overnight flight, you can ask for two things with absolute clarity: a sharp, alert, present, and quick mind to use to your advantage, and a kind, flexible heart full of regenerative feelings. By radiating this practice toward others, you not only activate the superior intelligence of the center of your chest, but this altruism also has a significant impact on your entire being. Above all, you'll experience better sleep, peaceful rest, and lucid dreams of exceptional clarity, full of information that comes from other spheres just for you, since generating feelings of appreciation and renewal toward others acts as a completely beneficial biological and spiritual key in your life.

Centralized egoism dissolves as your heart rate adjusts and your brain waves gently slow into a well-organized theta state of heightened awareness.

Every perception you have is linked to an emotion, and through this ritual you will be able to fully understand the high potency and potential you hold in redirecting your life. When you take ownership of your intuition, you begin to believe in it and learn to listen to it without a hint of doubt. You move from judgment to gratitude; discarding labels, you replace them with acceptance, and repetitive patterns transform into elevated choices.

This ritual is a great antidote to apathy, laziness, procrastination, and bad mood, as it allows you to see beyond your nose and register the interconnection you have with everything and everyone. By doing it at night, you become a luminous beacon that helps lost sailors reach a safe harbor and return home. You benefit yourself and others.

☆ RITUAL 38. VISIONARY

1. Lie down on your bed. Focus on the parts of your body that make contact with the mattress and the parts that make contact with the sheets or blankets. Breathe from your abdomen and identify an emotion or feeling that you want to change. Then, with complete sovereignty over what you feel and are experiencing, choose the one that will replace it. Be very precise in this

process. For example, if you have a tendency toward irritability, replace it with patience; if you want to stop complaining, replace your complaints with gratitude. Name the emotion you want to remove from your life and then name its replacement with clarity and forcefulness.

2. Activate the technique of focusing your attention on your chest and visualize your breath entering and leaving your heart. Feel your body relaxed in bed.
3. Begin to breathe the new feeling and emotion you have chosen to replace the one that does not serve you, and do so with great discipline in the process.
4. You have activated a center of complete vision, conquering mental delusions, stagnant ideas, and limiting thoughts, while cultivating a new relationship with yourself and your emotions. By practicing this ritual at night, you will enter sleep without unnecessary burdens or ruminating thoughts that keep you chained to suffering.

Purpose and How to Use It

You are a visionary and a pioneer in the art of managing your emotions by biohacking the habits that keep you repeating the same attitudes and patterns. You are successfully going beyond the obvious and apparent. This ritual opens you up to the power of discernment and peripheral vision simply by replacing a low-vibration tendency with one that elevates you and brings you joy.

What exactly is your "personality"? How do you define it? What words do you use to refer to yourself? We honor labels, becoming masters of portraying the assigned role—if we are told we are shy, then we retreat into solitude; if we are called rebels, defiance becomes our constant companion. . . . And so it goes, a cumbersome backpack overflowing with titles, adjectives, and nicknames.

This nightly ritual empowers you to hit the pause button. No longer will you be paralyzed by the flashing billboards that control you. Instead, you will access the power to replace those shadowy emotions with luminous and radiant ones.

Begin the replacement as if you were a surgeon removing a diseased organ, with total focus and determination, so that the change does not remain in the intellect or on the surface, but truly goes directly to your unconscious.

For example, if you feel helpless in complex situations and don't know how to say what you want, you can seek to transmute this state to a feeling of tolerance and maintain an open throat. Start breathing in the presence of the change you want to make until you truly reach a state of calm and the new feeling reigns throughout your body. Do not stop breathing and make the replacement until you have incorporated it fully; until your body and mind are in the tone of the new emotion and, when you close your eyes to sleep, you already carry this vision with you.

Until you achieve energetic change, you must continue your nightly practice. Your solitary bed is the best territory for expanding that inner consciousness. Keep in mind that, for some deeply ingrained attitudes, it is necessary to continue the practice for several nights in a row until the new habit has been established—you can continue with the same replacement for seven nights until you see great results.

Even if the seemingly negative attitude is justified (by your ego), try to get it out, because the emotional drain it produces does not justify the damage to your system.

Attitudes and emotions can be either renewing or draining. These emotional regulation strategies contribute to improving heart performance, increasing resilience, and accelerating recovery from stressors and trauma.

Self-induced positive emotions initiate the shift toward cardiac coherence and transform the addiction to suffering and stress into a new approach that allows you to build a reservoir of positive energy that you will explore during the night and will be highly beneficial for your day.

☆ RITUAL 39. ENTRANCE, EXIT, AND PARKING (4-7-8 BREATHING BEFORE SLEEP)

1. Stand beside your bed and envision the magical carpet on which you'll embark on a solo flight. With full awareness, step onto it and lie down with the intention of taking an initiatory and transformative journey. Visualize approaching an airport with three signs directing you: entrance, exit, and parking. You'll begin a three-part process using these images, employing your breath as an anchor before drifting into deep sleep.

2. Begin by approaching the entrance and inhale for four counts. Inhale through your nose, mouth closed. As you feel the air entering, mentally count four beats and simultaneously visualize how this new oxygen regenerates, opens, renews, and fills your body with green, luscious energy.

3. Now, enter the parking lot. Stay there paused, calm, and motionless, holding the air you just inhaled and counting mentally for seven beats. In this space of stillness, visualize that fresh, revitalizing air expanding through every pore of your body. Not a single space remains untouched by this oxygen.

4. At the exit area, you will release the air. Exhale for eight counts, using your vision to feel how your breath and its release carry away everything that doesn't serve you and is no longer needed, performing a total cleansing of your body. You have emptied everything, and it is time to start the cycle again.

5. Repeat this ritual for one minute (if you want to make it longer, do it for three minutes) and visualize the actions of arriving, parking, and leaving as your infallible allies before sleep. This visualization directly impacts your own circadian cycle, finely adjusting the balance between your sleep-wake states. In doing this ritual, you will be highly productive while maintaining an unprecedented calmness and peripheral vision that will allow you to see and hear subtleties shifting your existence.

Purpose and How to Use It

Just as at the entrance of an airport, where you are greeted by three arrows pointing you toward your destination, there are three key phases of your nightly journey. Simplifying these into three concrete, fundamental steps will help you achieve lucid dreaming quickly and effortlessly, and will support you in navigating the path toward your desired state without distraction.

First, an entry experience in which you inhale, allowing whatever you ask for or need to enter with your breath. Then an instant of pause, where you engage in a moment of conscious stillness, suspending the world around you and observing your thoughts, then the exit, where you enable yourself to release everything that does not serve for you, renewing yourself completely in the next breathing cycle.

Cycles that repeat themselves throughout existence and are manifested in highly significant events, such as births and deaths, or in subtle, almost imperceptible ways in the flow of ideas and emotions that are constantly in motion, both are reflected in that circular round of entry, parking, or exit.

This ritual is wonderful for reflecting on the pivotal moments in which you find yourself. You might feel like you're starting anew, at the entrance of something. Or, perhaps, you feel like you're in limbo, that seemingly nothing is moving, that everything is on pause. Or maybe you perceive yourself as leaving, letting go, releasing. Wherever you are, the use of visual imagery is a grounding wire that, combined with breathing, will begin a process of conscious oxygenation that will be absolutely new to you.

Additionally, the 4-7-8 breathing technique in this ritual calms the nervous system and, fundamentally, helps people with insomnia to lower cortisol levels, balance heart rate, soothe the mind, and lower brain waves to reach sleep in a state of deep meditation.

In your process of sleeping alone, you can observe, with much love for yourself, in which of the three stages you are, knowing that you can always start again. Honor your solitary bed as the territory of your own exploration, your own airport gate, from which you take off to evolve more and more each night.

☆ RITUAL 40. POWERFUL SLEEPING BEAUTY

1. As you sit on your bed, ready for sleep, begin a process of observation, taking in everything around you. Make sure to register as much as you can: textures (soft, rigid, solid, fluid), colors, and so on.
2. Once you have identified your surroundings and their qualities, soften your gaze by squinting until your vision is almost blurred while consciously focusing on the beating of your heart. In that position, gently move your eyes to the right, then to the center, then to the left, and then back to the center. As if saying "no" with your eyes, without moving your head. Repeat this five to seven times and then immediately relax and close your eyes.
3. Continue with your conscious and diaphragmatic breathing, visualizing the air entering and leaving your body as it travels down to your feet and rises to the crown of your head. Acknowledge any feelings that arise without interfering with or changing them.
4. Finally, bring your hands together at heart level in a prayer position and, applying gentle pressure to the thymus area, massage in a circular motion smoothly eleven times to one side and eleven times to the other, while continuing to breathe and connect with your heartbeat. Finish the process by lowering your arms and taking a deep breath in and out.
5. Now stretch, yawn, and surrender to the divine night.

Purpose and How to Use It

Within your mental, physical, and spiritual centers lie universes of subtleties that energetically reside within you and communicate with the surrounding cosmos, exerting influence over every aspect of your life.

Your body, your biology, is a perfect vessel where the balance of opposites, the generation of health and healing, and the awakening of light and consciousness depend solely on you and your commitment to your own cause. It is essential to understand how each of these parts is connected, united in perfect synchrony, so that you can break free from victimization, stop blaming others, cut off complaining at the root, and fully commit to an inner revolution that transforms your entire cellular environment into a high, loving vibration with your being.

This nighttime ritual has a clear and fundamental objective: to reach areas where a great deal of subtle energy is accumulated because, without the proper outlet and regeneration channel, it could produce a counterproductive effect of great emotional paralysis. With the movements of your eyes and the breath present in your heartbeat, you go directly to a sacred area of your physical heart: the sinoatrial node.

Nestled within the right atrium, the upper right chamber of the heart, lies the sinoatrial node—the body's natural pacemaker. This unassuming structure serves as the electrical conductor, initiating the rhythmic beat that sets the pulse. It generates an electrical impulse at a rate of sixty to one hundred times per minute, coursing through conduction pathways to trigger the contraction of the heart's lower chambers, propelling blood outward. As we transition into the realms of rest and sleep, this natural pacemaker aligns with the pineal gland, the orchestrator of melatonin production. This harmonious union paves the way for a night of exquisite rest.

This empowering ritual gently guides you along a somatic pathway, commencing with the gaze, observing the world that surrounds you. It then ushers you into a mystical practice of "seeing," softened by the movement of your eyes. You masterfully direct your breath toward your feet, consciously raising and lowering it. As you bring your hands together, massaging the center of your chest, you activate the thymus gland, responsible for T-cell production and the health of your immune system. More importantly, you cultivate awareness and connection with the engine of your heart: the sinoatrial node.

Embrace this sanctuary, the profound opportunity to transform into a powerful, conscious, and present sleeping beauty, one who wholeheartedly embarks on an exploration of the dream world, unburdened by the need for a prince charming to awaken you to grace and splendor.

☆ RITUAL 41. SELF-EMBRACE

1. As you lie comfortably in bed, begin by focusing on the gentle rhythm of your heartbeat. Take a few moments to center yourself, to fully experience this precious and uninterrupted opportunity for self-connection. It is recommended to do this ritual sitting comfortably, as this allows for a wider range of arm movement.
2. Cross your arms over your shoulders: right hand over left shoulder and left hand over right shoulder. Feel your hands resting gently on your shoulders and continue breathing from your abdomen.
3. Inhale and, as you exhale, begin to lower both arms simultaneously from your shoulders, passing through your forearms, elbows, lower elbows, and wrists, until your hands and fingers touch.
4. Repeat three times (or more, if it helps you calm down). Embrace yourself, whispering a soothing murmur with your mouth closed, all while gently swaying and humming a personal lullaby.
5. Continue breathing and notice the calmness it brings you, preparing you to enter deep sleep.

Purpose and How to Use It

This wonderful ritual confirms that you do not need external forces to soothe yourself. By crossing your arms over your shoulders, you symbolically traverse the body's midline, bridging the polarities and restoring harmony to neglected areas, giving yourself a hug. This act of self-embrace holds profound significance, for it marks the boundary between the upper and lower halves of your being, uniting the torso with the legs, the crown of the head with the pubis, the left and right sides, and finally, the back and front.

The self-embrace technique is based on the evidence that this intentional caress calms the brain, lowers anxiety and fears, brings the being back to its pure state, and generates a greater production of serotonin—a neurotransmitter linked to moods, which is key in balancing energy. Rubbing your hands slowly and caressing from your shoulders to your hands activates microreceptors in the skin that respond only to conscious and gentle touch, projecting calming information to the brain. The activation of these nerve endings is vital for emotional regulation and stress reduction, while inducing a process of deep and sustained rest and sleep.

The act of humming engages the centers of the mouth, tongue, throat, and saliva. This engagement triggers a cascade of neural activity, as crucial information is relayed from the nose and ears to the brain, culminating in a heightened state of consciousness. From this elevated state, you become the custodian of your well-being, nurturing yourself and activating your inherent power. You no longer need to seek external validation and you will feel, with full awareness, that producing these movements will balance and harmonize your entire immune system. You heal and expand the electromagnetic field of your heart; you are not a victim of invisible contracts that cause suffering. You hold freedom in the palms of your hands, and the loving message you send to your body is sealed during the night as you navigate the vastness of a darkness filled with mysteries for you.

☆ RITUAL 42. BIOLUMINESCENCE

1. Lie down comfortably on your bed, envisioning it as your magical flying carpet, ready to whisk you away once deep sleep embraces you. From this space, breathe and rub your hands together. Do this slowly and consciously, feeling each part you are touching. You can close your eyes to better connect with this experience.
2. Once you have activated your hands, run them over your entire body as if you were applying a rich, fragrant cream.

Again, be aware of what you are touching—each area, every fold—and accompany the movement and caress with your breath.

3. As you do this, invoke your bioluminescence and feel how your whole organism begins to glow from within. Each touch turns on the light of your skin, activates it, removes dead cells, and cleans spaces so that the brightness can appear in all its expressions.
4. Don't forget to visualize what's within you as well; that intelligent inner life that makes you who you are. Turn on the luminescence of your organs, tissues, bones, and muscles without neglecting the glands, blood, fluids, and internal systems.
5. Now that your body has been turned on, activated, and is shining, you are ready to go deeper. Turn on the luminescence of your heart by connecting, from the feet up, all the parts of your being.
6. Maintain the image of your luminous skin and repeat in a low voice, as you fall asleep: "I am a lighthouse. Light comes out of my pores."

Purpose and How to Use It
A symphony of life, this body speaks, listens, feels, perceives, and receives. Within its miraculous depths lie luminous opportunities, all beckoning to be embraced.

Within the sanctuary of my soul, a symphony of perfect intelligence orchestrates the dance of oxygen. These masterminds reside in my head, my heart, and my gut, yet their influence extends to every pore, every layer of skin, every chakra, and the vast network of seventy-two thousand *nadis* (subtle energy channels that carry oxygen, nutrients, and vital elements, creating an exchange highway in conjunction with the blood), ensuring my body remains in a state of pristine health.

Despite their variations and stories, all bodies function in the same way. We all have the potential to heal ourselves, detach from suffering, find the bright spots that sustain us, and hold the roots that intertwine with all and everything. We all have the opportunity to fly high, without limits.

Although we do not see it, we emanate light: we are bioluminescent beings, capable of emitting luminescence. Using a highly sensitive CCD camera, Japanese researchers Daisuke Kikuchi and Masaki Kobayashi at the Tohoku Institute of Technology discovered that the human body emits light. Though this light is too dim for the naked eye to perceive, it is powerful to know that we may perceive it with our other senses when we open ourselves to perception beyond matter.

The radiance we pour out is a thousand times below the sensitivity threshold of our eyes. It fluctuates throughout the day, influenced by our emotional states, thoughts, and physical condition. Our peak luminescence occurs in the early afternoon, gradually diminishing as night falls. The most luminous parts of our bodies are those most exposed to the sun, such as the cheeks and forehead.

On a physical level, our bodies emit light due to the interaction of free radicals with proteins and lipids, producing a faint glow. As a result, changes in our metabolism directly impact this bioluminescence. Emotionally, we shine brighter when we vibrate at a higher frequency—when we achieve coherence between our brain and heart, when we engage in acts of service, and when we recognize that our thoughts, actions, and words have a ripple effect on the world around us. This is why our luminosity increases when we sleep alone, as there is no exchange of other fluids, sounds, or chemical elements that accompany sharing a bed with another person.

The subtlety of this phenomenon is so unique and extraordinary that I wish you all the intention and focus to generate a great luminosity, knowing that during the night this will be an incalculable reservoir of rejuvenation and cellular reconstruction that will bring you healing and transformation.

CHAPTER SEVEN

LIMITLESS INTUITIVE INTIMACY

Immerse yourself in the realm of intimacy (derived from the Latin "intimus," meaning "deep," "innermost," or "at the core"). This is a sacred space, yours alone; it is a haven where you don't need to explain anything or justify yourself in any way. Here, joy takes on a solitary and profound quality. What voice would your intimacy have? What would it talk about? What would be its tone and rhythm?

Do you feel a connection with your intimacy? What are its colors and nuances?

These are challenging times for cultivating intimacy. It is difficult to find a place for it in the body and emotions when everything seems to scatter it, to prevent you from connecting with it or its messages. When everything is said, known, and exposed, the whirlwind of stimulation drowns out the solace of solitude's creativity. In this chaotic time when vulnerability is mistaken for chronic complaint and oversharing feels mandatory despite an alarming rate of superficiality, how can we rediscover the magic that unfolds in the uncharted depths of our own solitude?

The rituals in this chapter will assist, accompany, and guide you in the process of avowing your boundless intimacy. It is this unique and unparalleled intimacy that changes with you as you mature, taking concrete form in your process of assuming who you are, on the constant path of settling onto your queen's throne, while understanding and embracing the vastness of your existence.

There is an intimacy in true transformations—those that occur in the unconscious, sustained by lucid dreams, master mantras, an ear trained to sublime messages, and an innate ability to grasp perspective and detachment. Intimacy is united with intuition, because it is time to listen to both with great attention—to join them, to love them. The liberated space of the bed for you alone is the perfect territory for polishing your intimacy—the one that thinks big, without shyness, with supreme care for everything you feel and perceive.

Cultivate a practice of limitless, intuitive intimacy that awakens every fiber of your being. This intimacy resonates within you and radiates outward—a unique expression of your authentic self. Imagine yourself as a goddess, each sacred night in bed an opportunity for self-discovery and pleasure. Let these rituals be your guide as you reclaim your sensuality and explore the depths of your own intimacy.

☆ RITUAL 43. GLYMPHATIC CLEANSE

1. Begin by sitting down while breathing and feeling the weight of your head: its volume and the space it occupies. You can move it from side to side, make circles, activating its range of motion, and then, after a few moments, lie down resting it on the bed, with full awareness of the place it occupies.
2. Start at the back, the nape of your neck, and take a few moments to feel its presence. Notice how it sinks, which parts you feel more relaxed, what happens to the rest of your body.
3. Now, move it gently from left to right and from right to left, feeling your ears touch the pillow. Identify if there are any tensions and release them consciously, with the help of your breathing.
4. Rub your hands together and cover your eyes with your palms so that you begin to feel the play of lights, shadows, sounds,

and sensations that appear after these gentle movements.
5. Keep your eyes covered and visualize, using your imagination, the fluids; the liquid inside your brain moving in the form of lymph, which cleanses and carries away waste products.
6. End the ritual by surrendering to sleep, with the certainty that your brain center is detoxified, open to receiving messages from the universe in the form of lucid dreams.

Purpose and How to Use It

Your brain employs a flawless mechanism to purge toxic waste, expel the useless, carry away the accumulated, and discard the excess. It's called the glymphatic system, and just like your lymphatic system, it's responsible for maintaining your body's perfect balance, performing the magnificent task of purification.

Why is it crucial for night explorers to know, recognize, and honor this? Why is it so important when it comes to expanding consciousness and intuition?

It is during sleep that the glymphatic system activates, allowing waste products to exit, be absorbed into the bloodstream, and ultimately expelled from the body. The brain cleanses itself while you sleep, detoxifying and regenerating not only on a physical level, but also on an energetic one. Trash collectors come by and leave the bins empty; your glymphatic system releases what you don't need, opening up spaces for new things to enter while your lymph and its immune defense eliminate invading bacteria in a double mission to protect your being. All this happens while you sail on the magic carpet of your bed.

Your glymphatic system filters toxins from the brain that remain inactive during wakefulness, making sleep an unparalleled spectacle of the body's perfection and the organism's miracle. This unconscious intelligence takes care of absolutely everything without your conscious intervention in any of these processes. During this cleansing, a masterful transfer of frequencies takes place between your heart and brain. The sensitive energetic intuition is unveiled as the nervous system displays its artistry in detecting and responding to environmental cues. This gives rise to a new intimacy that goes beyond the expected and predictable, bringing you closer to the territory of a monk in a cave on a spiritual retreat.

This ritual recognizes and establishes you as the creator of your existence, while shedding light on a biological process with profound spiritual implications. Here, you become an active participant in this nightly cleansing, essential for your liberation.

☆ RITUAL 44. THE GRAND ALTAR OF YOUR INTUITION

1. Lie down on your bed and prepare for sleep, activating the absolute altar of your body. Breathe, rub your hands together gently, and bring them to the area of your uterus, two fingers below your navel. You will feel the warmth spreading as you rest your hands there, applying a slight pressure.
2. Begin massaging the area with both hands, counting eleven times clockwise and eleven times counterclockwise, breathing serenely.
3. While you do this, visualize an altar in your uterus, a space for your own expression in which you will place sacred objects, ceremonial offerings, prayers, and supplications. You can include any ideas or things that represent your spirituality and inner search, such as images, shapes, colors, as you are totally free to assemble your altar.
4. While you are massaging, begin to sing to this area of your body, setting a clear intention and putting out a high vibration to activate its power. Sing to it without shame or fear. Use the power of your voice to connect from your altar to the divine, in a double path of creator and created. Improvise, singing whatever comes to your mind.... Listen to your voice as if you were hearing it for the first time.
5. Now breathe from your uterus, just as you do from your heart. Lower your inhalation and exhalation to that area. Visualize the

air entering and leaving there as you organize your uterine altar to embark on the night's journey.

Purpose and How to Use It

Every mammal on Earth shares a profound connection—the nurturing embrace of the womb. This vital organ, cradled within the second chakra (*svadhishthana* in Sanskrit, meaning "house of sweetness"), is the strongest muscle in the body. It is made up of several layers of muscle tissue that go in different directions to make it practically unbreakable. Your uterus is incredibly flexible, as it can range in size from a pear behind the pubic bone to a giant balloon reaching the ribs and abdomen during pregnancy.

This organ is a source of healing and regeneration, as it generously and limitlessly produces stem cells during each menstruation to such an extent that scientists are studying the possibility of using menstrual blood to treat irreparable conditions such as Parkinson's, heart disease, and more, due to the vastness of its benefits. Your uterus is orgasmic, and it is extraordinarily connected to the universe in each female cycle. It is also linked to the movements of the Earth and the moon and to astronomy and quantum physics, which makes it an oracle if you know how to listen to it.

The uterus is the only organ in the body capable of nurturing another within, through the placenta, which provides the fetus with the precise nutrients it needs for nine months, and that is expelled at birth. The word *placenta* derives from Old English and means "a round, flat cake." As you can see, the tradition of honoring it continues to this day, as we celebrate each anniversary of our birth with a round cake, reminiscent of the sacred placenta.

Your uterus can nurture a human being within; it is a source of wisdom and sanity, it keeps you focused, it is your power center and your divine altar. From now on, during your nocturnal journey, you ought to give it the place it deserves. In the ritual, you must also sing to it, for when you do, it rejoices; it feels loved and recognized. The sound of your voice reverberates within its walls and opens spaces for new and wonderful things to come. If you want to create and believe, to understand and discover deep answers, practice this ritual on your uterine altar every night before embarking on your spiritual retreat, aiming for an unprecedented connection with your intuition.

☆ RITUAL 45. BENEFACTORS

1. Lying on your bed, close your eyes and feel the weight of your relaxed head on the pillow. Breathe as you visualize your benefactors; those who do you good, those who bring out the best in you. Bring them to the center of your heart and connect with each of their hearts.
2. Start with those who helped you during this day and acknowledge them as if you were looking them in the eyes. Remember who was by your side throughout the day—they can be people very close to you or even strangers who interact with you in a positive way. It can even be a sound or simply something you saw that opened your heart and helped you in some way.
3. Now, bring to your heart the constant benefactors who accompany you, help you, and are part of your life; those who are faithful, present; those who you know you can count on, no matter what happens.
4. In this step, elevate your vision and meditation to the invisible benefactors (they may be your teachers, ancestors, spiritual guides, etc.) who have or have had something to do with your life but are intangible. Gather them all to thank them for their constant care and the benefits that they bring to your existence.
5. Once you have the complete visualization, consider whom and what you benefit; for whom you are a benefactor. From a place of love, think of your role in the lives of others, the help and value they receive from you. Recognize yourself as a constant giver and benefactor and rejoice in it.

6. Finally, look at yourself as your own benefactor—the one who sows and cultivates self-love. Observe and embrace the benefits and wonders that you give yourself. Feel the emotions that arise when you reach this part of the ritual. Before going to sleep, remember to ask one of your benefactors to speak to you from the dream world.

Purpose and How to Use It
One of the fundamental thoughts and teachings of spiritual traditions (like Buddhism) is that everything we have, everything that happens to us, happens by the grace and kindness of someone else. Someone, something, a series of synchronicities and events have participated in your being here and now, in your holding this book in your hands, in life unfolding, in your breathing happening, in what you feel and how you vibrate.

We are all interconnected, parts of a grand tapestry woven from interdependence. Benefactors, those who have supported us on our journeys, have played a crucial role in bringing us to this path and allowing us to vibrate at this specific frequency. Their physical and spiritual sustenance has empowered us to rise above victimhood and transcend complaints. Recognizing and remembering these benefactors broadens our perspective beyond the ego's limitations. We begin to see ourselves not as isolated beings, but as participants in a vast cosmic plan.

Childhood wounds will fade away with ease, thanks to one or many benefactors who have brought you here, to this divine ritual that will make your intuition and intimacy with your heart flourish on a great scale. If benefactor identification proves challenging, return to your nightly visualization practice. Should the images waver, choose one that resonates most deeply. Let this benefactor serve as an anchor for your meditation, allowing you to feel the profound impact of their presence and its far-reaching influence.

The second step of the ritual delves into an introspection regarding your role as a benefactor to others. What is your influence? How do you exercise your leadership? What is the quality of your presence in the lives of others? How do you feel when you are recognized as a benefactor?

How do you manage clear and loving boundaries to give your best without feeling used or abused?

This ritual is profound, opening up questions that you must explore and navigate with courage and sincerity. Lean on writing; recording these emotions on paper is your grounding cable. Finally, as an exercise of deep spiritual intimacy, return to seeing yourself as your own benefactor, detailing what you need to give to yourself so that your journey is impeccable, whether you have to add things or, perhaps, remove some. How do you treat, talk, or benefit yourself? What decisions do you make to take care of yourself? Could you improve elements to be your own impeccable benefactor?

Complete the experience by invoking one of your benefactors to be present in your lucid dreams and, without fear, ask for what you need. The information you seek will be transmitted to you, without any doubt, in a clear and precise way.

☆ RITUAL 46. KEEP THE FAITH STRONG

1. Before sleep, stand still next to your bed for a few minutes, focusing on your heartbeat. Without moving, notice your feet on the ground, rooted to the earth, and follow the flow of your breath.
2. Raise your arms and bring both hands above your head, in a lotus flower position, as follows: join your hands and detach your index, middle, and ring fingers; leave only your thumbs and little fingers together. Open the separated fingers as if you were making a crown with your hands.
3. While breathing with your arms up, visualize your fingers and hands as antennas of loving, elevated forces, transmitters of celestial knowledge, spiritual certainties, and truths that only your heart knows.
4. Now, add a repetition or affirmation that you will say to yourself while your fingers, as extensions of your body, connect with the sacred that surrounds you. Start telling and repeating to yourself: "Keep the faith strong."

5. Repeat it seven times, "Keep the faith strong," and, as you do, register what you feel, where this phrase resonates within your body, where it feels most alive. Sense how it vibrates in your fingers and hands.
6. When you finish the repetition, lower your hands and arms, shake off any tension you feel, and get into bed, on the magic carpet between the sheets, ready for an uninterrupted nocturnal flight.

Purpose and How to Use It

How do you keep the faith strong? Where does this fundamental space reside that brings light to vitality and certainties, strength of your searches, and the serenity that anticipates decisions made from your inner power? This nightly spiritual retreat is a vast territory for the expansion of a consciousness that leads you to a place of total trust, of absolute surrender to what is happening, knowing that it is the fruit of your creative fullness. The kind of faith that moves mountains, of fervent religious people who simply trust and believe; that complete and total faith in yourself and in what sustains your existence is what you will cultivate in this ritual.

The longing for complete faith begins in this practice with your feet on the ground, feeling the base, your root, your connection with the earth; keeping your body active but relaxed, emulating a mountain that silently observes and feels. This is followed organically with the growth of the lotus flower (*padma mudra* in Sanskrit) over your head, facilitating celestial communication from above, which is distributed to your entire body and activates the purity of your heart as a symbol of the strength to prevail over obstacles and fears, to be reborn from the mud, and to keep faith strong despite everything.

The phrase you repeat to yourself has a powerful energy-opening effect; pronounce it with total conviction and firmness, almost like an order to counteract any doubt or distraction that crosses your mind. You say it, you listen to it, you keep repeating it until you feel that it flows through your veins and that your whole body understands and executes it. Esoteric principles, like those found in the mystical *Kybalion*, bring an initiatory and profound sense to the manifestation of high faith in all aspects of your life, because they offer a complete guide to the nature of reality. Its laws reveal the duality that governs the universe: everything has a counterpart, extremes converge, and paradoxes find reconciliation.

According to the book of Kybalion, the universe is a manifestation of cosmic consciousness where everything is in constant movement through vibration, and our thoughts have a very high power to shape the reality that surrounds us. The book beautifully explains seven laws that sustain the universe. Knowing and applying them will give you a map, a precise technology with instructions to spiritually understand how to achieve this state of strong faith.

The Seven Laws

1. **Mentalism**: All is mind; the universe is mental. The All is the totality. Nothing exists outside of the All.
2. **Correspondence**: As above, so below, as within, so without. This manifests on three grand planes: the physical, the mental, and the spiritual.
3. **Vibration**: Nothing rests; everything constantly moves and vibrates.
4. **Polarity**: Everything is dual; everything has poles; everything has its pair of opposites: like and unlike are the same; opposites are identical in nature, but different in degree; extremes meet. All truths are but half-truths; all paradoxes may be reconciled.
5. **Rhythm**: Everything flows, out and in; everything has its tides. All things rise and fall; the pendulum swing manifests in everything. The measure of the swing to the right is the measure of the swing to the left; rhythm compensates. The rhythm of your heartbeat is a key element in producing biological, emotional, and psychological alchemy.

6. **Cause and Effect**: Every cause has its effect; every effect has its cause. Everything happens according to law; chance is but a name for law not recognized. There are many planes of causation, but nothing escapes the law.
7. **Gender**: Gender is in everything; everything has its masculine and feminine principles. Gender manifests on all planes. On the physical plane, it is sexuality.

Remember the laws and keep the faith, confident that the power of your solitary night will integrate the opposites and smooth out the rough edges of emotional corners that you still need to heal.

☆ RITUAL 47. CLAIRVOYANCE

1. Sit on the edge of your bed with your arms relaxed. Open and close your fingers quickly to release tension. Breathing from your heart, bring the index finger of your right hand to your third eye, the point between your eyebrows. Apply gentle pressure so that you can feel it without discomfort.
2. Massage the area in a circular motion, clockwise and counterclockwise. Stay there, focused on the massage you are giving yourself while keeping your eyes closed and breathing. You can count eleven rotations to one side and eleven to the other.
3. While massaging this point, begin to ask. Ask for what you need, what you lack, what you hope will happen. Ask boldly, without shame or restrictions. Visualize what you desire and place it on your third eye, which you have activated with the massage.
4. Now visualize how your entire metabolism and emotions are perfectly regulated, helping your body and mind rest and make the most of your sleep hours. This opens a channel of absolute understanding.
5. From this place in your body, put yourself into orbit with masterful powers and see what is coming for you with total

clairvoyance. Write down the ideas and images that come to you, and then you can go to sleep.

Purpose and How to Use It

The center of clairvoyance, an inner eye that grants the ability to perceive the subjective intelligence of the unconscious and develop extrasensory and divinatory skills, enables the prediction of future events. Between the eyebrows lies the body's magical point, a powerful portal that, when touched, activates the cerebral zones situated in the brain's center. In Eastern traditions, this point is known as the *third eye*: the gateway that directly connects with the pineal and pituitary glands. Activating these glands opens channels of higher consciousness and intuition, allowing one to comprehend beyond the physical realm and enter a quantum field where the concepts of time and distance acquire an entirely different meaning.

Ancient Egyptians referred to the third eye as the "Eye of Horus" because the gland's structure not only resembles an eye but also, centuries later, scientists discovered that it possesses components similar to those of the eye, such as the cornea, retina, and lens. It is called the pineal gland due to its pine cone–like shape, which also symbolizes abundance and well-being. This shape can be found in many religions, from symbols of the Pope and Vatican to ancient embroideries and paintings. According to Vedic tradition, which predates Hinduism, the pineal gland is associated with the sixth chakra. In India, it is known as the "Window of Brahma"; in China, it is called the "Celestial Eye"; and Taoists refer to it as the "Niwan Palace."

This ritual effectively activates, cleanses, and decalcifies the pineal gland. In most adults, this gland becomes calcified due to environmental toxins, an unbalanced diet, lack of rest, a sedentary lifestyle, excessive fluoride in water and toothpaste, prolonged exposure to screens, and other factors. When calcified, the pineal gland loses its visionary quality from a mystical standpoint, slows down, and its intuitive power diminishes, disconnecting us from its guidance. From an anatomical and scientific perspective, this gland is responsible for producing melatonin, the hormone that regulates the sleep-wake cycle. If the pineal gland is inactive, the body's entire homeostatic balance is disrupted, leading to chronic inflammatory problems and diseases, depression, chronic stress, and other issues.

Activating the pineal gland is crucial because it unleashes a flow of clear and powerful intuition. You will no longer doubt the thoughts that reach your mind, or be swayed by external opinions. Rather, you will be centered and ask for what you need without hesitation. Great ideas will come to you with this ritual that opens a direct channel to your higher consciousness. During your nightly spiritual retreat, you nourish these ideas with sacred waters. Take advantage of the activation of clairvoyance practice before bed, as the lucid dreams you'll experience will surprise you, especially the level of response to your requests—everything you want and deserve you will receive.

☆ RITUAL 48. FIVE WISE ANIMALS

1. Moments before going to sleep, stand next to your bed. With your body relaxed but present, bring these five animals into your visualization: tiger, deer, bear, monkey, and crane. Notice the sensations each evokes, the imagery they stir within you, and the emotions they bring forth. Observe these responses without judgment, simply recording the inner landscape they paint.

2. Observe the tiger, the deer, the bear, the monkey, and the crane. Focus on their characteristics and dynamics and allow yourself to contemplate your own embodiment of these archetypes. Which aspects of your personality resonate with each creature? How do they intertwine within you? Which resonates most deeply? If you were one of them, what would you say? How would you speak?

3. Embark on a graceful journey of imitation, embodying the essence of each animal. For the tiger, extend your hands like claws, reaching upward with feline grace. Like a deer navigating the forest, sway gently from side to side, arms outstretched as if forming delicate antlers. Channel the bear's grounded energy,

swaying softly on your legs, shifting your weight with each gentle movement. Mimic the monkey's agility, stretching your arms as if swinging from branch to branch. Finally, stand tall like a crane, gracefully balancing on one leg and then the other.
4. When you finish the five movements, take a deep breath. Now you can go to bed and navigate in solitude in the most beautiful dream worlds you have ever seen.

Purpose and How to Use It
Ancient Chinese healers associated health, vitality, and balance with the practice of these movements derived from the ancestral system of qigong. In this ritual, I invite you to perform some magical moves to stir your stagnant energy before going to sleep, emulating the five wise animals of Eastern tradition.

For centuries, Taoist sages have observed and learned from these precious beings, mimicking their movements in the understanding that each one is related to the elements that give us life. Moreover, they are intimately intertwined with our emotions and offer us multiple energetic gifts. These creatures reflect strength, flexibility, power, vitality, and balance. By incorporating them into our movements, we integrate with their mysticism, activate unexplored memories of our animal kingdom ancestors, and move far more information from the unconscious than we can imagine. The movements of each one of them cultivate health and longevity, blood vessels open up, and we prevent diseases because we combine stretching, opening, and flexing, bringing harmony to all the energy systems of the body.

The creator of this system, the Chinese sage Hua Tuo, developed these routines to get to the root cause of disease. When you do these movements, imagine that each involved part of your body flows with the others, turning you into a cohesive and coherent being. Likewise, elegantly cross the meridians of your body (the highways of *Qi*, or vital force), bringing peace and confidence to all your cells.

In Chinese tradition, the tiger is associated with the gallbladder and works on the emotion of anger; the deer is related to the kidneys and bladder and works on the emotion of fear; the bear is related to the spleen and stomach and works on the emotion of worry; the monkey is the heart and small intestine and works on the emotion of joy; finally, the crane is the lungs and colon and works on the emotion of sadness. Therefore, visualizing them and moving to their rhythms shakes off what you don't need, prevents limiting and obsessive thoughts, and frees your being from the dark chains that have kept you tied to the same parameters for centuries. With great joy, feel like a tigress, a doe, a bear, a monkey, and a crane, and take these symbols with you on the night journey; of course, always adoring yourself in the process.

Let these power animals conquer you: allow yourself to be moved by them; let yourself flow, visualizing each of them and their mystical symbolism so that they appear within you as the pilots of your ship on the night journey. If you start dreaming about them or if they appear in your lucid dream, welcome them and write down everything you remember as soon as you wake up—they are messengers from a higher world.

☆ RITUAL 49. SOVEREIGN OF YIN

1. Begin by gently shaking your body at the foot of your bed, creating a vibration throughout your entire organism. Start slowly, allowing this movement to rise from your feet to the top of your head, expanding like a magnetic wave. Keep your lips and tongue relaxed so that the vibration reaches every part of your body.
2. Remember to breathe as you do this, so that you can combine the gentle rhythm of your movement to the timing of your inhalation and exhalation. When you feel that your whole body has been activated, stand up slowly, connecting with the beat of your heart in sync with your breath.
3. Now sit in a chair or on the bed and begin massaging the sole of your right foot, in the middle, with the pad of your left thumb. To locate the right spot, bend your toes slightly and find the crease. Repeat this massage on your left foot using your right thumb.

4. Make sure you do a counterclockwise circular massage. This is the most yin point on your body and this direction stimulates calmness. Continue massaging while breathing deeply; five times for each inhalation and five times for each exhalation.
5. Once you have completed these rounds, place your feet on the floor and notice how they feel. Shake your hands to release any accumulated energy and close the ritual by forcefully invoking the yin aspect of your sovereign being.

Purpose and How to Use It

The opposing yet complementary forces of yin and yang are present in everything. Ideally, they should be balanced; feminine and masculine energies in a dance (just like the famous black and white symbol of intertwined figures), always in equilibrium. When the natural homeostasis of our body occurs, we have a system in constant balance, free from abrupt accelerations that take us to the brink of the abyss or sudden stops that leave us confused and wounded.

To avoid being pulled in different directions, we flow in peace, bringing out the masculine part or the feminine part, as needed. An evolved consciousness is necessary to identify with total clarity what is required in each moment in order to become the sovereign of your yin, and feel your feminine aspect in full expansion.

For lucid dream experiences, conscious rest, inner development, and nocturnal spiritual practice in the retreat of sleeping alone, excess yang is one of the greatest holdbacks. The mind does not stop, thoughts are tumultuous, we ruminate on the past, project a catastrophic future, we walk without lowering our decibels, without taking a breath, always in action, in constant movement, doing without stopping, breathing mechanically. That is pure yang and it must be released and allowed to fade away so that the feminine, intuitive, and introspective part of yin begins to take center stage.

The ritual instructs you to move from the feet to the head in an upward spiral motion. Gently shake away the accumulated energy in your upper body, allowing it to flow through your feet and out into the earth.

Locate the midpoint of your soles, the gateway for releasing yang energy back to the earth. Imagine your bare feet connecting with the ground, visualizing the excess yang dissolving and disappearing, leaving the terrain fertile for your blossoming femininity: the embodiment of sensual and divine Venus.

This ritual is an act of high rebellion against a millennia-old structure that asks women to be productive, active, masculine, extroverted, and self-assured—the typical image of the "wonder woman" or "warrior" that has crushed yin energy and abandoned femineity in a dark corner. Here is your opportunity to bring it out and make it shine, especially so that your nighttime experience is unforgettable, and you are able to cultivate a corporeal and emotional intelligence that elevates you in your dreams.

CHAPTER EIGHT

WELCOME TO YOUR MAGIC CARPET

A woman's cunning and intelligence save her from her own death when she decides to tell her executioner a story each night; a tale that continues until dawn, never reaching its conclusion. It remains in suspense, leaving the fate of the characters and situations unknown.

The words "to be continued" flicker like a beacon. The man refrains from killing her because his curiosity about the story's outcome is stronger than his murderous instinct. Night after night, for a thousand and one nights, she engulfs him in her endless tale, weaving together stories, fables, anecdotes of lofty kingdoms, characters connected to the supreme source, soul alchemists, genies in bottles, magic carpets that transport the characters—unbeknownst to them—from universe to universe. A true marvel of quantum worlds, complex dimensions, interwoven tubular sacred geometry, elements that blend among sailors, beggars, spiritual masters, loving energies, and sexual passions.

Scheherazade skillfully ensnares Sultan Shahryar in Arabian nights of stories and legends, taming a ruthless beast solely with the power of her words. The story goes that the man killed all his lovers after a night of passion because he had once been betrayed by one of them and, driven by

CHAPTER EIGHT ☆ WELCOME TO YOUR MAGIC CARPET 141

this impulse, he murdered them without remorse. The man, masculine, a powerful king, and wounded in his pride (with a gigantic ego), found no other way to control women but to kill them. His vendetta knew no bounds; a trail of severed heads marked his path.

There is nothing new in what I am telling you: the immeasurable power of a woman is something so immense that if a man lacks conscience and humility, his only response to handle her is to put an end to her existence, making her disappear, humiliating her, hiding her, covering her body and her voice. However, with cunning, without rage, intelligently, using her heart as a guide, Scheherazade becomes a supreme symbol of the power of a woman who gently asserts herself and saves her life using her voice. The sound that comes from her throat, the inflections of the story and her unlimited imagination tame the sultan, who ends up surrendered with love and understands the greatness of this being that feeds him with fantastic stories.

The allegory holds true in all aspects of life. Ask yourself: who is your executioner and how do you tame them? Who is your sultan and how do you keep them at bay until you claim the power of love? Delve into these questions from your innermost being. The villain does not necessarily have to be a man or someone of flesh and blood, because in most cases you are your own assassin—the architect of self-deprecation and self-imposed limitations—blocking your light until the day you find your Scheherazade.

It's so beautiful when you let her come out and play! When you let her speak, dance, and show herself, to spread out without fear and conquer any obstacle. The Scheherazade that beats within you must show her attributes and gifts so that you can change your narrative and connect with your mission and vision without fear of headhunters and legendary refuters.

It is time for you to embroider and weave a new narrative, to climb without a seatbelt onto the magic carpet of your sacred and divine night.

☆ RITUAL 50. ACTIVATE YOUR *ISHINFURAN*

1. You can either sit on the throne (see ritual 6 on page 30 for a guide to creating your throne) next to your bed or choose to go straight to bed. Sit down and breathe from your stomach,

touching your heart with your right hand. Feel the beat and its rhythm.
2. At the same time, touch your forehead with your left hand and register the tensions in your body. Remember to keep your shoulders away from your ears so that oxygen can circulate without interruption.
3. Breathe simultaneously through both hands and through the areas they are touching, as if the air were entering and leaving through these anchor points that connect you to your body.
4. While continuing this breathing and with awareness of the physical sensation of your hands on your heart and forehead, add the repetition of the Japanese word *Ishinfuran*. When you inhale, say it in your mind or aloud. Repeat it also when you exhale.
5. Continue with the ritual until you feel calm, and then you can release your hands and shake them out.

Purpose and How to Use It

The Japanese concept of *Ishinfuran* means "when the heart and mind are in the same place." With soul and mind, brain and heart, and undivided attention, activating this word within you is essential to fully experience advanced states of grace and feeling the body in fullness.

When you say it, its own vibrational quality appeals to the unity of all parts. When you pronounce it, you make a pact of self-love and self-care through a deep connection with your sacred magnificence.

Like our heroine Scheherazade, tamer of dangers with her words, this ritual allows you to get rid of low-frequency verbs and adjectives and enter the major leagues of mind and heart in coherence. Remember that the journey on the magic carpet is accessible and free, but you must create the right weather conditions for the flight. If the sky is stormy, the pleasure of the flight will be clouded by your tense body; on the contrary, if you activate the Ishinfuran process, you can let yourself be carried away by the starry cosmos of the divine night without alterations or anxieties. Listen to your voice, pay attention to your inner dialogue, and be firm in your decision not to feed suffering.

This magical word is an anchor to prevent you from straying from your purpose. Just this one change in your narrative can completely alter the course of your life. The fragile and established "reality" in which you live is merely a product of your perception, based on habits and choices. Therefore, it is your decisions that lead you to paradise or hell in a matter of seconds. When you hold the keys to your own process, you realize that every moment holds immense purpose: your power of choice becomes your superhuman ability. Immerse yourself in connecting with your Ishinfuran so that heart-brain coherence and this transformational axis become your guiding light as you embark upon lucid dreams on your magic carpet.

☆ RITUAL 51. EMBRACE OF THE THREE GATES

1. Find a comfortable position and sit on the bed. Close your eyes and start breathing while bringing your right hand to your left side, at rib level.
2. At the same time, move your left hand and hold the back of your right elbow. Each of these parts fits perfectly with the other, so that you are totally comfortable and relaxed.
3. Take a few slow breaths and reverse the position—left hand touching the ribs on the right side and right hand touching the back of the left elbow.
4. When you have repeated this for five breaths on each side (at least), breathe again a few times until you feel true calm. Lower your arms and remain serene as you enter your bed, ready for sleep.

Purpose and How to Use It
This self-embrace embodies an ancient technique for calming and grounding those powerful emotions that leave you feeling overwhelmed and confused. We need to lower their volume, soften their shrillness, redirect them, and reinvent them. This embrace activates three key energy centers

in the body: the upper center, encompassing the brain, heart, and lungs (the humidity chamber); the middle center, encompassing the liver, kidneys, stomach, pancreas, and spleen (the maceration chamber); and the lower center, encompassing the small intestine, colon, bladder, and sexual organs (the drainage chamber).

In traditional Chinese medicine, this meridian, called *Sanjiao*, "three chambers or three spaces," is the one that governs our body's ancestral response when we face violent situations or stressors: we freeze, defend ourselves, or flee. By establishing this embrace at the points of the ribs and elbows, synchronized with your breath, you organically and integrally soothe the meridian, sedating the stress response in the body and thus minimizing its impact on your overall well-being. Once again, you return to yourself, to your enormous capacity for self-healing, activating the internal pharmacy that resides within you. Here, collaboration, not competition, guides your evolution and thought processes. Your thoughts, ideas, and moments of insight play a vital role in maintaining your holistic health.

You can create your magic carpet on your sheets to take flight in the world of dreams. Completely devoid of fears, you can let yourself be carried away in total surrender to the experience, generating the perfect space both inside and out in which to navigate. Breathe through your triple embrace, in these three sections of your body, as you elaborate your infinite flight plan.

☆ RITUAL 52. SELF-OVATION

1. Before sleep, give yourself an ovation next to your bed. Applaud, celebrate, and cheer yourself on to the highest degree.
2. Begin slowly, feeling the entire palm of your hand, fingers, spaces, and the friction between the parts as you initiate the applause ritual.
3. Visualize your triumph, your success, and everything you desire and need manifested in all its power. Increase the speed of your applause while breathing, identifying how your heartbeat accelerates.

CHAPTER EIGHT ☆ WELCOME TO YOUR MAGIC CARPET   145

4. "Hack" your mind by changing bad habits for productive ones, and making better decisions. Repeat while applauding: "Standing ovation for my being. I deserve this. I applaud myself!"
5. Without judgment or interruption, record the thoughts and emotions that arise during this ritual. Check if your mind defaults to self-criticism or if you instead feel a sense of comfort and belonging.
6. After a few minutes, ease into a slower tempo, then stop and shake your hands, sharing the energy you have generated to the universe. From this state of self-love, imagine yourself on a podium, then gently lay your head on the pillow and surrender to sleep.

Purpose and How to Use It

Have you ever stopped to applaud yourself? To give a standing ovation to your existence, just like you would to your favorite artist?

Give Yourself an Ovation.
Give yourself an ovation.
Applaud yourself.
Applaud yourself.
Adorn yourself with laurels.
Put on your medal.
Step onto the podium.
Start your fan club.
Give yourself an ovation.
Give yourself an ovation.
Adorn yourself with laurels.
Put on your medal.
Step onto the podium.
Start your fan club.
A standing ovation for your being.
Give yourself an ovation.

Give yourself an ovation.
A standing applause for your being.
Shout it from the rooftops.
Communicate it.
Put it on social media.
It's time to applaud yourself.
You deserve everything.
A standing ovation.
Acknowledge yourself, admire yourself.
A standing applause for your being.
For your being.

All acts of self-celebration have been condemned by religion, education, and other imposed schemes, making it impossible for you to feel the joy of honoring yourself. Yes, you alone, without anyone to organize your celebration or be your audience; the wild and beautiful act of asking yourself to sing and dance; of hanging a medal around your neck and accepting a prize while applauding yourself. That is what this ritual invites you to do, to the rhythm of bachata, as if you were giving yourself a private party for your own existence.

Moving self-love energy is your task; no one will do it for you and activating this intention before entering a lucid dream is one of the most powerful things you can do. Not as an intellectual idea, but as a poetic act for yourself.

During your lonely night, feeling the pleasure of sleeping alone, you will fly on the magic carpet, and your energy will be connected to joy, the deep certainty of your supreme existence that deserves to be shouted from the rooftops and given a standing ovation. Use this ritual to celebrate: by applauding yourself, you are generating happiness hormones, moving stagnant energy, activating meridians of the hands that connect with each other when they are touched, expanding your own sound, and returning to your ancestral origins—when we danced and sang around the fire in a tribe.

With a round of applause, a new instrument emerges: your voice. For applause and singing naturally go hand in hand. As you establish the ritual of self-applause, you'll find yourself singing in no time. Step on the gas, even if your mind tries to sabotage you and make you stop. Keep applauding yourself until you become your own biggest fan, your own rock idol, your own favorite actress. This astral journey on your solitary bed requires a great deal of happiness and joy, and this ritual is the key to generating it. Step onto the podium, open up the fan club, and . . . sweet dreams!

☆ RITUAL 53. SEEKING NOCTURNAL REFUGE

1. As you lie in bed, before drifting into deep slumber, take a few moments to breathe and visualize a refuge. What does this haven represent for you? What form does it take? Is it a place, a person, a situation, or a moment in your life?

2. With complete presence, seek refuge, protection, care, and attention. Begin by seeking refuge in a higher being, a divinity in whom you believe. Say, "I seek refuge in . . ." and name them.

3. Now, seek refuge in nature; in the forces of the sun and the moon, in the directions and elements that make you human. Speak your words clearly, requesting this protection.

4. Seek refuge in your community, your friends, your family, and your loved ones, whether they are living or not. Seek refuge in the wisdom of your ancestors and their miraculous resilience that allows you to be alive and remember them. Name each and every one of those to whom you direct your request.

5. To complete the ritual, seek refuge in yourself—your higher self, your understanding and wisdom, your qualities, and your aspirations. Say your name and seek refuge with absolute certainty that you can grant it to yourself. Now you can surrender to sleep with the confidence that you will be absolutely protected and cared for on your nocturnal journey and in whatever happens upon awakening.

Purpose and How to Use It

We have not been taught to ask. We have been conditioned to be givers, to always be available, to be the refuges of our relationships—families, coworkers, pets, everyone. Asking for refuge is a sublime act of spiritual growth that involves breaking many habits and imposed frequencies, because it takes you out of a small and constrictive view of the world and of yourself. In Buddhism, one of the main practices is to take refuge in three elements—the Buddha (the superior being), the Dharma (knowledge), and the Sangha (the group, peers), feeling them in the heart, without any doubt that one day we will reach enlightenment.

The pronunciation of the words and the request in this ritual immediately condition your mind, body, and spirit to receive something new; to find a different experience in everyday life, performing this conscious act that generates feelings of compassion toward yourself. This enormous and beautiful compassion has nothing to do with guilt, shame, or complaint, but rather stems from the deep feelings of protection, refuge, and care that you have the right to ask for.

Visualizing these beings in whom you take refuge creates new neural connections, lowers stressors, and educates you in the fine-tuning of your requests so that what you need is clear and precise. It also facilitates that, during sleep, you can understand yourself more and more. It is a prayer, a plea that does not come from books or classes, but that you create yourself. Lubricate the stagnant areas; areas where you feel that energy is not flowing, and is therefore preventing you from having a more beautiful waking experience, and journey on the magic carpet.

Ask and it shall be given. Speak your needs and, as the words leave your lips, transformed into breath, they materialize. Share your stories and ask your questions, but above all, make your requests without shame. For this practice in the sanctuary is not merely to make you feel better or calmer; it is to radically transform your perception of yourself and your relationship with the world. Through it, you will gradually emerge from the illusion of ignorance and enter the territory of the novice apprentice of freedom.

CHAPTER EIGHT ☆ WELCOME TO YOUR MAGIC CARPET 149

☆ **RITUAL 54. THE HEART'S SMILE**

1. Stand beside your bed with full awareness of your feet on the ground. Inhale slowly while raising your arms and hands upward; make sure that the inhalation corresponds with the moment you raise your arms for coherence and synchronization. When you raise your arms, imagine that you are filling yourself with life, air, total renewal, and that you take everything you need.
2. As you exhale, lower your arms and hands slowly, with your palms facing your body, while making the sound "heeeeeeeeeeeee" for as long as your exhalation lasts.
3. At the moment of release, imagine heavy, stagnant, confused energy leaving through your hands toward the ground. Return what no longer serves you in an act of instant self-cleaning.
4. Repeat the practice seven times, feeling how your mind and body relax with each breath and how, with each inhalation and exhalation, you let in what you need and release what needs letting go.
5. When you complete the seven rounds, bring your hands to your heart (I recommend the left hand touches your chest and the right hand covers it). Breathe from the center of your chest, imagining a big smile in that area of your body that grows with each beat.
6. Inhale and, each time you release the air, produce the sound "haaaaaaaaaaaaaaaaaa" for as long as your exhalation lasts. Visualize that this sound opens the frequency of your heart's electromagnetic field. You can immediately rest your head on the pillow and prepare for a wonderful solo sleep. Enjoy!

Purpose and How to Use It

Sound is the essence, the profound source of healing and creation; it's the most advanced medicine that you create and produce solely with your voice. It is a symphony of high-frequency vibrations that resonate within every cell of your being. Your body's energy centers are invigorated to embrace a life of well-being, unburdening themselves from the shackles of repetitive narratives of discomfort and constant guilt. Meanwhile, your mind is engaged in a novel endeavor, not orchestrated by intellect, but by the wisdom of your heart.

As you produce these sounds during the ritual, in harmony with your breath and movements, you are incorporating two expansive waves with a transcendence that goes beyond reason. These waves will awaken your unconscious mind, inviting the boundless world within you to take center stage in the most spectacular dream flight you can imagine.

The ritual commences with the resonant sound of "heeeeeeeee," a vibration that harmonizes and balances the internal organs intimately connected to the vagus nerve. With each repetition, your heart and lungs expand, your digestive system reaches an optimal temperature, and your pelvic region relaxes, fostering a profound connection between the cervix and larynx. As you move your arms and breathe while emitting this vibration, the upper part of your body opens to a deeper understanding, enhancing self-awareness and purpose. Joints lighten, detoxify, and de-inflame.

In the second phase of the ritual, the sound of "haaaaaaaaaaa" awakens your heart's innate melody. As you release this vibration, your heart's electromagnetic field expands, radiating an immediate surge of well-being throughout your body. The utterance of "haaaaa" guides your mind to the central channel, the channel of the heart, fostering positive thoughts and initiating devotional chanting. Pronouncing "haaaaaa" prompts your heart to smile; this expression and its vibration trigger a physical shift, transforming your heart into a beacon of joy, fully aligned with your well-being.

Your movements and what comes out of your throat become the rudder of your magic carpet. Both will guide your experience so that it becomes unlimited and incomparable; the night journey of your soul takes you to territories full of answers, luminosity, and a new way of loving yourself.

☆ RITUAL 55. *VIPARITA KARANI MUDRA*

1. Find a comfortable spot on your bed to lie down with your legs extended upward, resting against the headboard or a wall. Elevate your legs effortlessly and maintain the position for a few minutes (5–7 minutes is ideal).
2. Remain in this position, breathing deeply. You can rest your arms alongside your body or place your hands gently on your abdomen. This is the perfect moment to practice some of the mantras from chapter 3. As you lie in this posture, you will feel the circulating blood in your legs shift and change due to their elevated position, with the soles of your feet facing the ceiling.
3. Once you feel completely relaxed and your legs have reenergized, slowly lower them back down, assume a horizontal position, and surrender yourself to sleep.

Purpose and How to Use It

Inverting oneself, turning upside down, changing position, elevating what is normally below, reverting functions, stepping outside of narratives where things are always the same; these are some of the benefits that this yoga pose, as ancient as the first texts of this discipline, brings to your body, mind, and spirit. In Sanskrit, *viparita* means "upside down" and *karani*, "in action"; therefore, the pose reverses and balances fluids and, with that, it collaborates with the journey of prana, or vital energy, in all the channels of your body. Mentally, it offers a new perspective; literally, you can observe your legs and feet from a different point of view, like you're walking on air. With your legs up and your head down, you can open your wider vision to discover a surprising world.

As we defy the body's natural order, viparita allows new and oxygenated blood to reach the upper extremities, stimulating the passage of lymphatic fluid that cleanses and rebuilds, sweeping away bacteria and parasites from your blood. Additionally, it releases pressure from the lower back, gives vital space to the kidneys, and heals inflammation and fluid accumulation in the feet, ankles, and legs. Not only are you putting your lymphatic system to work properly, but the glymphatic system also benefits (see ritual 43 on page 124), since, by bringing your legs up and having your head down, you contribute to a cleansing process that will happen during sleep.

In this way, you become a reservoir of expanded consciousness—an active collaborator in the processes of your unconscious world and your autonomic nervous system. As you relax in this position, your breathing inevitably slows down and communicates to your vagus nerve that you feel safe and calm. Therefore, your parasympathetic system, responsible for calmness and balance, is beautifully activated, sending positive and loving messages to your brain, throat, heart, and diaphragm. It even reaches your intestines, thus connecting your three intelligence centers. Being both a pose and a *mudra* (symbol or gesture that elevates the subtle body's energy), it is a divine tool with which to raise your vital energy, break free from melancholic and depressive states, and step onto your magic carpet without fear.

Warning: This pose is not recommended if you are menstruating, pregnant, or have high blood pressure. Enjoy it very much when you do it!

☆ RITUAL 56. THE LIGHT OF THE WORLD

1. In your room, with your bed prepared for the most pleasant journey of your life, light a candle and place it near you.
2. Allow the candle to illuminate the darkness and make sure it is the only light you have around, so that you can truly feel its effect.
3. Breathe and register your thoughts and emotions as you observe where this candle is reflected within you.
4. Visualize the light of your higher beings, spiritual masters, guides, or gurus emanating from the candle and ask them to show you the paths, to give you signs, to manifest.
5. Before going to sleep, look at the light so that it remains on your retina. Ask for guidance and the appearance of the light frequency in each part of your being and your life. For your lucid

dreams, you can anticipate the appearance of this light so that it expands to all those who need it. The light is not only for your benefit, but also for the benefit of those around you.

Purpose and How to Use It

The symbolism of light holds immense power (you can combine it with ritual 5, *Trataka*, on page 28). It encompasses everything from the simple flame of a candle to lamps, lights, or lighting systems, representing the emergence from darkness. It also symbolizes the optimism of clarity at the end of a tunnel and the victory of clearness when the veils of the mind and heart are lifted. The candle, the flame, the fire; associated since the dawn of humanity with consciousness and the ability to hold the light of life, hope, creativity, and connection with the divine. This is why candles are protagonists in all temples, churches, and places of prayer, as they remind you of your true essence and, at the same time, represent the birth of an idea, the divine spark in the search for the path of authenticity.

In this ritual, harness the flame as your inspiration and focal point. Through its radiant glow, invite the companionship of your higher guides as you embark on a nocturnal journey of heightened consciousness. Within your lucid dream, invoke a call to your higher self, your limitless potential, the embodiment of your deepest aspirations. Allow the external light to ignite your inner flame for, by intertwining these paths, you steer your conventional mind in a new direction. Transcend the realm of concepts, venturing into an abstract, boundless, and unpredictable realm, where mysteries await.

As you soar on your magical carpet, let your glowing candle illuminate the path before you. Become a beacon of hope, radiating light not just for yourself, but for all beings you encounter. In this way, your journey transcends personal awakening, fulfilling a mission to spark the light of awareness in slumbering hearts.

Warning: To ensure safety, consider using a battery-operated candle that can remain lit throughout the night, avoiding any fire hazard.

CHAPTER NINE

SOVEREIGN OF THE BED AND YOUR LIFE

Stellar Vibration
You are stellar vibration.
Inner understanding.
Manifestation of the whole.
An expanding mystery.
A story without an end.
A spiral of light.
A spaceship.
A party, a dance, a handmade drum.
A box of surprises.
The one who speaks without words.
A mystery manifested.
A celebration.
You are everything you dream of.
You are pure eternal light . . .
You are that and more.

CYNTHIA ZAK
"VIBRACIÓN ESTELAR" (STELLAR VIBRATION)
FROM *ENCIENDE TU CORAZÓN* (IGNITE YOUR HEART)

CHAPTER NINE ✸ SOVEREIGN OF THE BED AND YOUR LIFE

Oh, sovereign queen, you who embrace all emotions with a vow of unwavering presence within yourself. You are that stellar vibration that resonates, "My song, the cosmic vessel, a mortal who transcends mortality." You are all of this and more, and now is the time to shed the limitations and embrace your grandeur in its fullest expression and expansion. Kiss the ground that supports you, breathe blessings to your left and right, ask for what you need, trust that you are not alone. What appears to be reality is merely an acquired system of perception, and everything can be changed if you venture into the forest's embrace and become wild.

Before you lies a precious human rebirth, something unique and hard to achieve, for among millions and trillions of incarnation options, you have been granted the gift of being human and being a woman. Do not squander this gift; etch all your desires into the agenda of the air and earth, water and fire, and clearly express what lies within your chest, within your heart. Draw lines of light between your womb and your brain; between the triangles above and below that form a Star of David. Begin to imagine a triangle with its apex at your third eye and its vertices at your shoulders; simultaneously create another with its apex at your pubis and its vertices at both points of your hips. In the space between your two inverted triangles, where your heart and internal organs reside, visualize a circle connecting them. The Star of David is a talisman of protection and divine connection that opens paths for you in all directions.

Open the windows and adjust your peripheral vision to encompass all the details surrounding your focus, for there lie the answers. Create your altar, craft your *stupa* (a Buddhist symbol representing the mind), and circle it repeatedly in constant prayer, so that joy may never depart from your being. You are healing yourself and you will heal seven generations past and seven to come; you are doing it.

With your left foot firmly planted on the ground, initiate a graceful spin like a whirling dervish, arms outstretched toward the heavens. Reach high with your right hand, palm open to receive, and balance with your left hand extended downward, ready to give back. Remember, everything is an exchange of energy. This is how you undergo transmutation—a profound shift that begins at the very core of your being, the very essence of your genes. The ancestral inscriptions etched in your blood are rewritten, paving the way for something grander, something boundless. Embrace this transformation with full consciousness, acknowledging the yearning that has led you to this moment.

Engage in a meticulous cleansing ritual, washing away any negativity. Bless your food with gratitude. As you cross thresholds, hold the intention of leaving suffering behind, for your actions hold the power to liberate many from such burdens. Craft new narratives, weaving stories that ignite your spirit and keep you on the precipice of dawn, yearning for ever-deeper knowledge with each passing night. Allow these stories to silence your inner critic, so that the pure love within may shine brightly through your actions, emotions, and words.

Fill yourself with curiosity, open yourself to the mystery, and embark on a mission of maximum renewal, a silent revolution of mythical proportions. Finally, enter your sacred bed, your magic carpet of power. Find joy in your solitary nights, a spiritual retreat that follows the lunar cycle. Nourish your intuition, that inner knowing that feels and senses even when words fail. Experience all this in a flow of heightened consciousness—a state attainable only when your mind, emotions, and heart are in sync.

☆ RITUAL 57. THE DERVISH

1. Enter your nocturnal sanctuary, a realm of solitude and absolute freedom. Stand before your bed, placing your hands on your heart, feeling its rhythmic beat, activating the flow of oxytocin, the love hormone. Remember to always place your left hand on your chest, gently covered by your right.
2. Applaud yourself for being here, in this moment, with the clear intention of connecting with your most spiritual essence before drifting off to sleep.
3. With your hands still resting on your heart, pose the questions: "How do I envision myself in the future? How would I

feel in a new reality?" Project your desires as if they are already unfolding, expressing gratitude in the present tense. For everything you desire is already happening now, not in the future. Fill your mind with words that evoke elevated emotions and amplify the smile of your heart.

4. Engage in conscious breathing. Extend your right arm, palm facing upward, as if receiving a gift from the heavens, like plucking an apple from a tree. Keep your arm slightly extended, hand open with fingers gently curled.

5. While your right hand receives, your left hand faces downward, giving back to the earth. This symbolic gesture represents the perpetual exchange of receiving and giving. Maintain this posture of your arms and hands as you breathe, counting seven complete breaths (each complete breath includes one inhalation and one exhalation).

6. Between your outstretched arms, your solar plexus and chest area become accessible and open. You can visualize and feel your heart pulsating at the center, as this posture fully exposes the thymus channel (located in the center of the chest), allowing a pathway of unconditional love to flow through this region.

7. With arms outstretched, initiate a gentle rotation. Keep your left leg firmly planted on the ground, serving as your axis. Counterclockwise, raise your right leg, simultaneously generating momentum from your hip. Pivot on your left axis two or three times, maintaining outstretched arms and a steady gaze on a fixed point to prevent dizziness.

8. Perform the previous step again slowly, two or three times, feeling the rhythm of your heartbeat, the expansion of your arms receiving and giving, and your body producing a circular motion that supports your rest process from the balancing center of your brain. After these rotations, gradually come to a standstill and remain breathing calmly until you feel ready to surrender to divine night.

Purpose and How to Use It

A *dervish*, a mystical seeker of oneness with all, is a spiritual practitioner with an unwavering resolve to shift their assemblage point, rewiring their neural pathways to manifest a new reality in their body, emotions, and approach to life. To be a dervish is to be a mystic of grand proportions, focused on polishing the veils of the heart and mind to perceive beyond; to break free from a lukewarm, comfortable existence while remaining firmly anchored to the earth. You can soar and enter altered states of consciousness yet remain rooted in the here and now, your body in pure communion with all of existence. Beginning with the heart and heightened emotion, you infuse this intention into your arms and hands, which symbolically encompass all—receiving and giving; giving and receiving—in an unceasing dance.

As you touch your heart, oxytocin, the love hormone, awakens. Feel what happens in your raised right arm—the open line extending from the center of your chest down the left side—transforming your upper quadrant into an upward-pointing triangle receiving divine light from your crown. Here, the heart serves as the intermediary between the higher worlds (mental and spiritual) and the lower ones (physical planes). From the waist down, an inverted triangle extends to your feet, which begin to move in a whirling motion, emulating the primordial condition of your existence. In this condition, everything revolves: atoms, the blood within your veins, the solid and soft structures of your body; they are in an unconscious revolution, which you bring into conscious awareness through this ritual.

You are engaging in a profound meditation; a practice of immense subtle power that regenerates your brain and creates a new pathway from the vestibular area of your ears to the rest of your head, simply through the movement of your arms and legs. As you flow in this rhythmic dance, your body receives enhanced oxygenation, effortlessly connecting you to planets and solar systems that accompany your rotation. Practice this meditation whenever possible.

Enrich your movement with a gentle murmur (refer to rituals 10 and 24 on pages 40 and 80), a soothing sound. Produce this murmur from your tongue, moving it toward your larynx and pharynx, to instantly calm any emotional disturbances. This practice effectively extinguishes the flames of negative emotions that hinder your well-being.

Prepare your body, mind, and spirit to channel the vibrant energy of a whirling dervish. Allow this divine dancer to emerge within you—to swirl, twirl, and revel in the transformative experience as your dormant *kundalini*, life force, awakens, igniting a surge of vitality and spiritual awareness.

☆ RITUAL 58. THE *SEPHIROT*

1. Lie comfortably on your bed, preparing for this powerful ritual. Begin by bringing awareness to your body, starting with the right side, from the sole of your foot, paying attention to each toe. Slowly move upward, focusing on your calf, knee, leg, torso, and arm, including your fingers, palm, and back of the hand. Continue to your shoulder and the entire right side of your face.

2. Repeat the same process for your left side, ensuring you don't miss any part: on the left side of your body, starting from the sole of your foot to each toe, move up your calf, knee, and leg. Similarly, scan your torso and arm, including your fingers, palm, and back of the hand. Continue to your shoulder and the entire left side of your face.

3. Now, visualize and scan the midline of your body, the line that perfectly divides both sides, starting from the sacrum toward the crown, from bottom to top. Perform this with utmost consciousness, ensuring you don't overlook any part or detail.

4. Once you've completed scanning the sides and the midline, scan your entire back, starting from your feet, legs, glutes, back, nape, and head. Visualize your body as a tree with its roots, trunk, and branches filled with leaves, flowers, and fruits.

5. Use this mantra as an affirmation, repeating to yourself: "I am the tree of life, I sustain life." Once you've completed it, breathe peacefully and surrender to deep, restorative sleep.

Purpose and How to Use It

The practice of conscious body scanning stands as one of the most profound and transformative tools for connecting with your unconscious world. As you systematically connect with the physical sensations of your body, you embark on a journey of redefining your self-perception and opening a spiritual portal from your physical realm.

As you bring your body into sharp focus while lying in bed, visualizing yourself as a tree, glimmers of higher forces descend upon you, interconnecting you with a profound and elevated knowledge that transcends mere intellect. This wisdom springs forth from every cell of your being, an exquisite nocturnal poem that aligns you with the kabbalistic Tree of Life. The Tree of Life is composed of ten spheres or Sephirot, each embodying ten attributes and ten creative forces through which the Creator reveals itself with its infinite power to create and sustain our world.*

The tree mirrors your body divided into three parts: your right side represents the principles of unity, harmony, and benevolence; your left side, the realm of power and strict justice; and the midline is a symbol of perfect balance.

Just as each part of the tree serves a unique purpose and must work in harmony for it to be fruitful and healthy, so, too, do your mind, body, and spirit form a perfect triad, unifying wisdom and compassion.

The Tree of Life serves as a roadmap for connecting with your inherent sovereignty, guiding you through ten manifestations that resonate within. The challenge lies in fully integrating these aspects to transcend a fragmented existence and embrace wholeness.

The ten sacred wheels or components of the Sephirot represent your inherent attributes. Beginning at the crown, *Keter* embodies the connection to your creative mind, the grand spirit, and the concept of a universe guided by light—a force far greater than yourself. Approach your crown with humility and certainty, inviting blessings, wisdom, protection, and benevolence.

Descending to your right shoulder, *Chochmah* represents wisdom, the

---

*The word *Sephirot*, from the Hebrew תוריפס, singular *Sephirah*, means "emanations, radiations." A Sephirah is something that shines.

CHAPTER NINE ☆ SOVEREIGN OF THE BED AND YOUR LIFE

flashes of inspiration that illuminate your path. With unwavering faith, call upon this area when seeking knowledge and clarity.

On your left shoulder resides *Binah*, the embodiment of understanding, the transformative power that converts abstract ideas into tangible realities. Seek guidance from this area when pursuing the fulfillment of projects and dreams.

At the center of your chest, level with your heart, lies *Da'at*—the confluence of wisdom and understanding. This pivotal point holds the key to manifesting your desires, while simultaneously serving as a profound reminder of your heart's intelligence, akin to a brain within itself. Seek guidance from this inner oracle, for its response is unwavering, never misleading or faltering.

Aligned with your right rib cage resides *Chesed*—the embodiment of kindness, benevolence, and expansion. These fundamental elements nurture your feminine power and provide the anchor that balances hyperactivity with the need for rest. Gently touch this area, seeking clarity and direction.

Opposite Chesed, at the level of your left ribs, lies *Gevurah*—the source of strength, sound judgment, law, and power. This energy creates a harmonious equilibrium with its counterpart.

Within the realm of your uterus, the altar of your body, resides *Tiferet*—beauty, truth, and the central channel of the Tree of Life. This point serves as the bridge between heaven and earth, a wellspring of compassion and balance between the upper and lower areas.

Upon your right hip resides *Netzach*, empowering you to conquer obstacles and achieve resounding victories. In harmonious balance, *Hod* graces your left hip, safeguarding the glory and divine splendor that permeate your very existence.

Before reaching your legs, the midline of your body culminates in the pelvic and genital region, known as *Yesod*. This is the base and mystical connection between giver and receiver, connected to all other channels and bringing forth life.

Finally, your legs and feet represent *Malchut*—the source of the physical world, these grounding roots absorb the essence of the earth, providing nourishment and stability. The lines that unite the ten points symbolize the connections between the different levels of the cosmos. No part or section is more important or better than another, as all cocreate equally, providing a map that marks the path for everything that exists.

The Tree of Life isn't an external or distant, abstract concept. Your body is the tree: your essential self is this set of permanent interconnections where every part corresponds to a powerful, invisible world waiting for you to acknowledge it and ask for everything you desire.

Nourish your Tree of Life during the night. In deep and lucid sleep, everything that appears will be a ceremony of encounters with these ten luminous spheres that inhabit your being.

☆ RITUAL 59. NOCTURNAL WILD SIDE

1. Settle into your bed, acknowledging your emotional and physical state. Breathe deeply, letting go of anything that weighs you down. Before drifting off to sleep, make a list of wild things you'd like to do or experience. Don't hold back on your fantasies—let your hand write freely, without thinking.
2. Write from your unconscious mind using free association. This means one word sparks a cascade of meanings, images, and memories that you put on paper to manifest. Let your writing take shape as you express yourself.
3. Build your "wild" list. Include new plans, ways to talk to yourself you've never tried, sexual experiences swirling in your head, wild trips, spiritual awakenings—any desire you want to acknowledge. Write without judgment, whether it's realistic, achievable, or pure fantasy.
4. The first thought is the right one. Follow what pops into your head first, don't let your mind sabotage you. While making your list, connect with the joy and excitement of exploration.
5. There's no length requirement for your list. Write what feels right for you. Tuck it away before sleeping. After writing your wild fantasies, consciously register what happens during your

CHAPTER NINE ☆ SOVEREIGN OF THE BED AND YOUR LIFE

sleep and then look for signs throughout the day that confirm what you put down on paper.
6. Repeat this ritual for as many nights as you like. The key is to let yourself flow, without interfering with your wild list. You'll be amazed by what emerges from your forgotten inner world, now becoming a source of life and energy.

Purpose and How to Use It

I'm not here to suggest anything specific. Instead, I invite you to loosen the metaphorical scarf that's been tightly wound around your neck for ages. Remember the untamed spirit you once embraced? The raw, unfiltered version of yourself? Recall the symphony of the forest, the crackling fire painting the night sky, the ability to navigate in darkness without a lantern, guided by your feline instincts. Do you remember that feeling of anonymity, blending seamlessly with the trees, free from the constraints of shoes and phones? Relive the days of roaming music bands, solo backpacking adventures, assembling circus tents, or hitchhiking down every alluring road. Can you summon memories of naked days, tarot readings at dawn, drum skin washings in the river, passionate lovers, or misty shamanic covens? Can you still smell the Ganges, feel the wisdom in its waters, or hear the muezzin's call to prayer? Do these memories ignite a spark within you? A time when boldness and radiance defined your every step, each one a blossoming miracle?

A wild spirit has no room for suffering; it leaves no space for guilt, let alone complaints. A wild woman doesn't waste time blaming others for her feelings, words, or experiences. Instead, she takes the reins of her mind and activates the command center in her heart. A wild spirit liberates the protagonist from the pain stored in her muscles, transforming her into an open channel for knowledge from heaven to earth. Tension melts away from her shoulders, her joints release their burdens, doubts are embraced and nurtured for a while, and then gently released.

The wild spirit sings in Sanskrit, unconcerned with the meaning of the words. It is the vibration and the sacred experience of opening the throat, allowing these ancient syllables to dance upon the tongue and emerge on the breath, that truly matter. The wild spirit gazes into the eyes, unfazed by the judgment of others. She holds the gaze with an audacious defiance, inviting others to shed their societal lenses and decipher the depths hidden within the irises of their fellow beings.

Above all, the wild spirit cannot be swayed by the notion that her thoughts and feelings are wrong or inappropriate. Her aura exudes such tranquility and strength that the opinions of others simply do not register. Realigning one's life with joy takes precedence over all else. Victory, enigma, soul harmony, elegance, beauty—a portal to mysteries envelopes this wild spirit. Inspired by the solitary embrace of the night, she carries this wealth into her waking hours, infecting those around her with this divine state where anything is possible.

☆ RITUAL 60. REPAYMENT

1. Throughout the day, gather items that hold significance for you, representing a token of appreciation, a repayment to the Earth. These could include flowers, petals, fruits, seeds, spices, tobacco, incense, feathers, crystals, stones, sweets, written words on paper, and so on.
2. Before drifting off to sleep, assemble these elements, arranging them into a mandala on a paper napkin. Approach this task with mindfulness and attention to detail, as if adorning the most opulent palace.
3. Wrap your offering like a precious gift, securing it with a ribbon. Encase it meticulously, as if it were a jewel, and place the mandala beside your bed to absorb your nocturnal energy. Embrace the emanations of your chosen objects, each carrying a sacred energy that will accompany your intention for a lucid dream during the night.
4. In the morning, seek out a patch of earth, a flowerpot, or a corner where you can bury your mandala with its offering. Ensure that all your selections are biodegradable, as you will be entrusting them to the earth with the firm intention of making

CHAPTER NINE ✦ SOVEREIGN OF THE BED AND YOUR LIFE 165

a payment to the planet that so generously sustains you. Dig a hole in the earth and gently place your wrapped napkin containing your offerings.

5. As you cover it with earth, sing, pray, chant, recite mantras, or blow gently, offering your breath in gratitude to every corner of the Earth.

Purpose and How to Use It

Returning to the Earth all that it gives us is a profound act of self-love, and the ritual of repayment accelerates our awakening processes like no other. From the moment we select offerings, an internal transformation unfolds. Ego falls away, replaced by a new worldview. Repaying Earth is an act of supreme spiritual transcendence that deeply impacts our psyche and emotions. It symbolically represents the greatest act of gratitude to the Great Mother, shaking us free from apathy and ruminating minds, bringing us back to the only thing that matters and exists: this present moment, as we wholeheartedly celebrate the Earth that nourishes and sustains us without asking for anything in return.

We pay, return, give, and gift, and each element we offer in our ritual carries our attention and intention. We return to our heartbeat and the intelligence of our hearts to choose the offerings that we will bury later, as the vibration of our soul must be tangibly manifested in each of them.

To do this, take your time and carefully consider the items you'll offer. Choose elements that hold personal significance and resonance with your life experiences, transforming your offering into a portable altar. Imbue your napkin with this magical energy, and as you bury it, enliven it with your breath, song, and the rhythm of your respiration. I recommend making an offering at least once a month. If it aligns with your menstrual cycle, even better. For those who don't menstruate, synchronize your offering with the lunar cycles, choosing the full moon phase.

The chosen location can remain the same each month or vary depending on your preference: all you need is a small patch of earth. Ensure that the items you bury are biodegradable (no plastic, please), as these offerings will become one with the earth, nourishing its depths. Each offering can be unique, reflecting your current experiences and emotions. Remember that the elements need to have profound symbolic power and carry a high vibration, in order to leave an enduring imprint on the planet. Sugar signifies sweetness, flowers or seeds represent tenderness, and combining these with fruits or vegetables conveys the nourishing essence of these foods as an offering to Pachamama, Mother Earth.

Approach this ritual with an open heart and a receptive mind, for its power is undeniable. The act of burying your offerings opens a deep channel of humility—your hands become soiled as they touch the earth; the minerals and vitamins from Mother Earth enter your pores, balancing your electrons and protons. Additionally, you must lower your head, bending down to acknowledge that without this nurturing soil, life cannot be sustained.

You stand in the presence of the Mother, the Virgin, the Teacher, the Creator, Protector, and Bestower. Kneeling before her, your hands gently touching hers, you initiate an interstellar communication, weaving a new tapestry of connection. For you know that Pachamama, the Mother Earth, holds your secrets close, processing and transforming them into seeds of renewed ideas, awakening your consciousness to a broader worldview that places you as an absolute pioneer of your own life.

Embark on this ritual when you seek solace amidst painful or traumatic experiences, or use it to celebrate life's triumphs, offering gratitude in the very place where these blessings unfolded. Approach it with mindfulness as you close chapters, bid farewell to houses or spaces, and embark on new journeys—to new homes, careers, or lands where you can sow the seeds of your dreams. Bury your offering and, as night falls, bring it to mind before drifting into the first stage of sleep. Remarkable revelations await you.

☆ RITUAL 61. PLATO'S CAVE

1. Take a deep breath and light a candle. Sit on the edge of your bed, positioning yourself to observe your shadow's reflection on the wall in a meditative state. Regard this phenomenon with detachment, without labeling or judging. Always

CHAPTER NINE ☆ SOVEREIGN OF THE BED AND YOUR LIFE 167

remember to return to the rhythm of your heartbeat as your compass and guide.

2. As you breathe calmly, establish a conscious connection between this image and the shadows that inhabit your thoughts, emotions, and mind. Consider your dark side: your secrets, fears, anxieties, and limitations that prevent you from breaking free from your current state. Your shadow on the wall presents an opportunity to identify the shadows that reside within you.

3. Acknowledge these shadows, but do not attach yourself to any of them, nor dwell on the narratives of suffering they may evoke. Simply observe them, and with all your intention, begin to blow. If a shadow emotion arises, blow on it. Literally, inhale and exhale, releasing the air until it dissipates. You'll notice how they quickly dissolve because they lack substance. They are merely reflections, not your true self.

4. Register, without judgment, the frequency with which you confuse shadows with who you are, and how the dark discourse in your mind gains significance, even though none of it is happening in reality. These shadows are just your mind repeating a learned script, a vicious cycle that makes you addicted to suffering.

5. Observe, again without judgment, the influence and intermingling of others' shadows with your own; how they seek to become a part of your existence, even if you haven't invited them. In this moment, decide that they will leave your being definitively, never to return. They belong to their owners, for you no longer believe in their reflection, in their mirages, but rather seek the true depth of your soul.

6. Once again, blow away any remaining lingering shadows and shake yourself from head to toe. Now, fully prepared, surrender to your lucid dream, seeking guidance to discern between those who offer hollow forms and those who nurture your spiritual growth.

Purpose and How to Use It

Plato's Allegory of the Cave paints a vivid picture: prisoners chained and immobile, forced to stare straight ahead. A fire blazes behind them, casting flickering shadows on the wall before them. These shadows become their entire reality, the only world they've ever known. None of them have ever considered that these are mere reflections of forms, lifeless flickers devoid of substance. They believe these shadows to be the true essence of reality.

Trapped in this world of shadows, they are convinced that these are the only things that exist, utterly certain that this is the entirety of the world, that nothing lies beyond. They settle for what they know, unable to perceive anything else. In this parable, Plato introduces a hero, an initiate who begins to question everything until he manages to escape and emerge from the cave. At first, the sunlight blinds him but, as his eyes adjust, he comprehends what has been happening. Even with his damaged vision, he begins to perceive a different aspect of reality. He discovers that they have been deceived, that they have only seen shadows—a fragment that is only the reflection the guards want them to see. Upon his escape, he encounters the vast universe, the open air, nature in all its splendor, and his true capacity for adaptation and joy.

The liberated prisoner returns to the cave, bursting with newfound knowledge and a burning desire to save his companions, and that is when he gets the complete notion of the wall, the fire and the shadows. Driven by urgency, he starts removing their chains. However, to his surprise, the prisoners resist, they consider him a madman, unhinged, dangerous, a mass agitator, a revolutionary; they believe there are insurmountable dangers outside, that the sun will blind them, and they decide to remain in captivity. They prefer the chains to the challenges and wonders of freedom. Fear of the unknown overcomes any hint of curiosity about what life would be like beyond the shadows.

There are hundreds of interpretations and perspectives on the allegory of the Greek philosopher, but the one that matters in this ritual has to do with life in the cave, the influence of others, and the discernment between light and shadows. The cave is a symbol of the passage

CHAPTER NINE ☆ SOVEREIGN OF THE BED AND YOUR LIFE

between the upper world and the lower one; a space preserved from the light where there are other rules of the game. The lower world is a territory often compared to the womb of the Earth and the mother, which shelters and protects, but that at some point must be abandoned to live and breathe on one's own.

In the depths of darkness only shadows are visible, and the illusion of a projection masquerades as reality. This calls for a deeper exploration of the influences in your life—who you follow, who shapes your perceptions, your choices in groups, people, relationships, and friendships. If the entire group, like the cave dwellers, fears liberation, where does that leave you? Who do you listen to and follow? Who are your guides and teachers? When someone arrives from the outside with a fresh perspective, an unconventional way of living, and invites you to break free from the cage, how do you respond? The most crucial step is to break free from the self-inflicted shackles of self-flagellation, where you become your own captor, silencing and restraining yourself. This happens every time you allow a limiting thought to fester and grow until it becomes a reflection on the wall, a looming presence against which you feel powerless.

Within you lies a magician who yearns to escape the chains; there's an ever-present opportunity for liberation. From this moment forward, your commitment is to remove the gag, dispel the shadows, and challenge the status quo that paralyzes you with fear. Embark on the ascending path, even if the initial burst of sunlight blinds you. The dream world and the passage of your being through the stages of sleep offer an extraordinary launchpad for this ritual. Seize this opportunity to seek deeper insights, to grasp the whole picture rather than fragments, to expand your understanding of yourself and your existence. Let the messages you receive during the night illuminate your path from the cave toward the light.

☆ RITUAL 62. THE RAINBOW

1. Lie down comfortably on your bed. Breathe slowly and deeply, bringing the image of a rainbow to mind. Think about it in detail: its colors, its shape, the space around it, the times

you've seen it in the sky. Ask yourself how you feel when you see it and what thoughts come to you.
2. Now create your own meditation using these four steps. Bring them to mind in this order:
   - Look at the rainbow.
   - Notice its perfect curve.
   - Pay attention to the colors.
   - Watch it fade away, consciously observing it as it disappears from the sky. Be aware of how it vanishes.
3. Repeat this sequence three times, focusing on your heartbeat and breathing. Once finished, allow yourself to drift off to sleep. Take the physical feeling of a great release, based on letting go, with you as you enter the sacred night.

Purpose and How to Use It

When you witness a rainbow gracing the sky, a surge of joy fills your heart. You capture it in photographs, perceiving it as a phenomenon brimming with messages for you. It symbolizes a sign, a calling, a moment of pure delight. You understand that in mere moments it will vanish, yet this realization neither saddens nor troubles you. You are fully immersed in this gift of nature, and letting go of it causes no anguish. On one hand, you recognize that you are powerless to retain it; on the other, you acknowledge that the rainbow's fleeting nature is an intrinsic part of its essence. Thus, with the knowledge that other rainbows will follow, you release it without sorrow or clinging. Or do you find yourself lamenting its departure?

Attachment is the primary culprit behind neurosis, sadness, pain, stagnation, depression, and other emotional turmoil. Its antithesis, detachment, serves as the most potent and transformative force for inner liberation and growth—an indispensable element on the spiritual seeker's path. This deeply poetic ritual offers a remarkable practice to begin discerning how these opposing forces resonate within you, how they manifest in your life. How often have you experienced a sense of

CHAPTER NINE ☆ SOVEREIGN OF THE BED AND YOUR LIFE

rebirth, despite initial fear, when you made the conscious decision to let go and release?

As you embrace detachment, releasing and relinquishing with wisdom and compassion, and stop forcing things, a fundamental law begins to take root: the law of receiving, of being gifted, bestowed upon, open to surprises, of allowing yourself to be loved and cared for. With the intelligence of your heart, you come to understand that everything that unfolds in your life is a product of your own choices; as you open yourself to experiences in new territories, welcoming what comes your way, you learn to ask and use your voice as a guiding path. Just as in the meditation of the rainbow, the gift comes to you: you savor and enjoy it, yet you let it go without regret or resentment. Detachment becomes your guiding principle, your way of life.

We cling to concepts, ideas, judgments, opinions, material possessions, people, and countless objects. Releasing these attachments, letting them go, emptying our closets, giving away furniture, separating from partners, bidding farewell to children, embarking on new chapters, and flowing with change without drama proves to be a daunting task. Most challenging is the detachment from preconceived notions, labels, and prejudices that have been deeply ingrained since the beginning of time, forming a hardened plastic mold around our minds and hearts. Unless we make a conscious effort to expunge these limiting beliefs, they will continue to constrain our lives.

Detachment begins within ourselves; it's a task for our minds and emotions. Only we have the power to sever the ties that bind us, to step out into life, and to silence the internal voices—the constant self-dialogue reinforced by the opinions of others regarding what we should do, say, and think.

As you prepare for sleep, envision a rainbow in your head. Just as its vibrant hues fade, your consciousness begins to surrender, transporting you into the uncharted and enigmatic realm of dreams. Embrace detachment to relinquish control over your body and allow yourself to soar on your magical carpet, never knowing where it might take you.

☆ RITUAL 63. MEMENTO MORI

1. Rest your head on the pillow. Breathe deeply, bringing your hands to your beating heart, and remember that you will die.
2. With heightened awareness and profound respect for your life, place a hand on your heart and the other on your womb. Remind yourself that you are here but fleetingly.
3. Continue breathing, honoring this present moment; your body on the bed, the sacred night, the doors of mystery that you will enter once you drift off to sleep, and remember, once again, that you will die.
4. Sink into the bed, release all tension, and surrender to sleep.

Purpose and How to Use It

You chose to arrive in this form, in this body, in this time and space, in the place where you were born, and with the family that you selected. Your mind has been migrating for millions of years, and even your bones contain stardust and cosmic elements from other galaxies. You have passed through countless states—you were a mineral, a plant, an animal, and now, the master of your perfect human rebirth. No one knows when or how, but the certainty of death's inevitability touches us all; no one has walked away from this Earth alive, and that's why the meditation on remembering death is the most important thing you can do for your life.

This remembrance that the end will come is your great engine of enthusiasm and purpose, ensuring that your passage through this world and each of your breaths are not in vain. You always desire to find a way to honor your existence and the existence of everything that surrounds you. Make the most of every moment, and get into your magic bed—your ship, your carpet—with full presence and joy, because the moment you close your eyes and your consciousness begins to soar, you have the opportunity to experience death more closely.

For ancient cultures, death was not thought of as the end. Rather, it was considered a stage; a transformation with which the soul flies to reincarnate again and again until completing a cycle. With this poetic view, you surrender to meditation and the memento mori ritual, so as not to waste a single moment in destructive internal dialogues, in relationships that drain you, in things that do not serve you, or in people who suck your energy.

Memento mori is the recognition of life's impermanence: the engine that ignites your passion for living fully, your ecstasy, your answered prayers and fulfilled desires. Embrace impermanence—you are a tenant in this body, and your greatest transformation awaits.

Navigate in your solitary bed with a full smile, trusting and celebrating your breathing with the supreme awareness of the knowledge that you will die.

☆ *LANIAKEA*: THE FINAL RITUAL

The universe is a vast cosmic tapestry woven with an unimaginable number of galaxies. *Laniakea*, meaning "immense heaven" in Hawaiian, is the name of the supercluster of stars that makes up our universe, consisting of approximately one hundred thousand galaxies.

Within this grand expanse, you and I are connected by this book and its rituals, our hearts beating in unison on the Earth—just another planet in the universe. Look up at the sky and let your gaze ascend toward the heavens. Here we are, floating in the vast and infinite universe, a grain of sand with immense power, knowing that beyond this precious blue dome, there is nothing . . . or is there? Be profoundly aware that you are on this vessel sailing through the cosmos, surrounded by galaxies in transit through Laniakea. Expand your soul and heart with deep gratitude for being a part of this frequency. Here and now.

> As you lie down to rest, review your day from beginning to end in the greatest detail possible. Before drifting off to sleep, ask for what you desire without hesitation or fear: remember to create your motivation. As you rest your head on your pillow, use the last moments of wakefulness to let go, activating detachment and

perspective, for all that you have witnessed has become a part of the past: it is over. You can view what has transpired as a movie in which you played the lead role, but you have the opportunity to change and improve as many times as you wish. This marvelous practice is fundamental for cultivating a heightened sense of gratitude and self-love. As you do so, always follow the rhythm of your heartbeat so that the fire of your heart remains ablaze throughout the night, never to be extinguished.

It is my greatest wish that these rituals become your constant companions, transforming into your sacred geometry for attaining clarity and certainty, illuminating your days and nights. May you find joy in their practice, unwavering faith in your infinite power, and may your nightly spiritual retreats be productive, enriching, and captivating. With each practice, may you witness the transformative power within your mind, your vibration, and your thoughts.

To my fellow solitary sleepers, I'll meet you here. The journey is in your hands. Enjoy it!

REFERENCES

American Academy of Sleep Medicine. "Over a third of Americans opt for 'sleep divorce'." Survey. Atomik Research Agency, July 10, 2023.

Atkinson, William Walker. *The Kybalion: A Study of the Hermetic Philosophy of Ancient Egypt and Greece*. Chicago, IL: Yogi Publication Society, 1908.

Better Sleep Council of the United States. "Sleep and Partners Research 2023." Better Sleep Organization website, March 31, 2023.

Borges, Jorge Luis. "El sueño." In *El otro, el mismo*. Buenos Aires, Argentina: Emecé, 1964.

Bower, Bruce. "The Oldest Known Grass Beds from 200,000 Years Ago Included Insect Repellents." Science News, August 13, 2020.

Braun, Adee. "The Once-Common Practice of Communal Sleeping." Atlas Obscura, June 22, 2017.

Carney, Colleen, and Rachel Manber. *Quiet Your Mind and Get to Sleep: Solutions to Insomnia for Those with Depression, Anxiety, and Chronic Pain*. Oakland, CA: New Harbinger. December 2, 2009.

Cook, David. "Mysticism in Sufi Islam." *Oxford Research Encyclopedia of Religion*, 4 (May 2015).

Coveney, Catherin, Michael Greaney, Eric L. Hsu, Robert Meadows, and Simon Williams. "Contextualizing Sleep." In *Technosleep: Frontiers, Fictions, Futures*. Surrey, UK: Surrey University, 2023.

Dell'Amore, Christine. "Chimpanzees Make Beds That Offer Them Best Night's Sleep." *National Geographic*, April 18, 2014.

Fick, Franklin. *Five Animal Frolics Qi Gong: Crane and Bear Exercises*. 1876.

Holt, P. M., Ann K. S. Lambton, and Bernard Lewis, eds., *The Cambridge History of Islam, Vol. 2: The Further Islamic Lands, Islamic Society and Civilization*

Jung, C. G. *Dreams (from Volumes 4, 8, 12, and 16 of the Collected Works of C. G. Jung)*. Translated by R. F. C. Hull. Princeton University Press, 2010.

Ledger, Sally. *The New Woman: Fiction and Feminism at the Fin de Siecle*. Manchester, UK: Manchester University Press, 1997.

Lyons, Malcolm C., and Ursula Lyons, trans. *The Arabian Nights: Tales of 1,001 Nights: Volume 1*. London, UK: Penguin Classics, 2008.

Mallison, James, and Mark Singleton, eds. *Roots of Yoga*. London, UK: Penguin Books, 2017.

Paulson, Genevieve Lewis. *Kundalini and the Chakras: A Practical Manual—Evolution in This Lifetime*. St. Paul, MN: Llewellyn Publications, 1998.

Plato. The Republic. Vol. 4 of Dialogues. Madrid: Gredos, 2003.

Richardson, Benjamin Ward. *Vita Medica: Chapters of Medical Life and Work*. London, UK: Longmans, Green, and Co., 1897.

Schutz, Manon Y. "Mighty in Waking and Great in Sleeping: The History of Beds in Ancient Egypt." Presentation, Essex Egyptology Group, April 2, 2017.

Sismondo, Christine. "Should We Normalize Sleeping in Separate Bedrooms? Experts—and Frustrated Couples—on the Booming 'Sleep Divorce' Trend." Health and Wellness. The Star website. January 15, 2024.

Wadley, Lyn, Christine Sievers, Marion Bamford, Paul Goldberg, Francesco Berna, and Christopher Miller "Middle Stone Age Bedding Construction and Settlement Patterns at Sibudu, South Africa." *Science* 334, no. 6061 (Dec 2011): 1388-91.

Wangyal Rinpoche, Tenzin. *Tibetan Yoga of Dream and Sleep*. Ithaca, NY: Snow Lion Publications, 2011.

YeYoung, Bing. "Origins of Qi Gong." Sacramento, CA: YeYoung Culture Studies, October 17, 2011.

Zak, Cynthia. *Enciende tu corazón, 77 rituales*. Buenos Aires, Argentina: VR Editoras; Mexico City, Mexico: VR Editores, 2021.

Zisapel, Nava. "New Perspectives on the Role of Melatonin in Human Sleep, Circadian Rhythms and Their Regulation." *British Journal of Pharmacology* 175, no. 15 (2018): 3190-99.

INDEX

4-7-8 breathing, 115–17

Activate Your Ishinfuran ritual, 141–43
Aho Mitakuye Oyasin, 64–66
alpha waves, 18, 99–100
altruism, 73
amygdala, 20
anger, 98
animal liberation, 46–48
applause, 144–47
arboreal sleep, 9
astral bodies, 74
astral journey, 9
attachment, 170–71
attention, 2
autonomy, 11
awareness, 2

baby boomers, 12
basal forebrain, 20
baths, 7–8
beds, 3–4, 8–10, 10–12, 22–23, 37–38
   Cardinal Points ritual, 27–28
   Conquering the Bed ritual, 24–25
   Encounter With Your Guru ritual, 23–24
   Oneironaut ritual, 25–27
   Sit on the Throne, Queen ritual, 30–32
   Speak Softly to Yourself ritual, 32–33
   Trataka ritual, 28–30
Benefactors ritual, 128–30
beta waves, 18, 99–100
Better Sleep Council, 4
Bioluminescence ritual, 120–22
birth, 58
blankets, 23
blood pressure, 16, 74
body temperature, 13, 15
Borges, Luis, 91–92
brain, 19–20
brainstem, 19
brain waves, 17–18
Bright Mind, Kind Heart ritual, 111–12
Buddhism, 51

Canada, 13
candles, 29, 153
Cardinal Points ritual, 27–28
Carney, Colleen, 13
cause and effect, 133
Cerebral Pathways ritual, 42–44
chakras, 70–75
chi, 37
circadian rhythms, 11–12, 14–15
Clairvoyance ritual, 133–35
Clear the Right Nostril ritual, 94–96
Clitoris ritual, 85–87

coherence, 108–11
communication, 73
compassion, 107
Conquering the Bed ritual, 24–25
correspondence, 132
cranial bones, 43
crown chakra, 74
crowns, 31

darkness, 4
death, 58
delta waves, 18, 100
Dervish ritual, 156–59
detachment, 98, 171
detoxification, 43
discernment, 13
dream yoga, 94–96
drooling, 40–42
duty, 11–12

earth element, 38
East, 28
egoism, 112
Embrace of the Three Gates ritual, 143–44
emotional body, 14
emotions, 112–14
Encounter With Your Guru ritual, 23–24
Entrance, Exit, and Parking ritual, 115–17
Eroticism Everywhere ritual, 87–90
expansion, 74
Eye of Horus, 74, 134

face, 88
faith, 130–33

feng shui, 36–38
fire element, 37–38
Five Wise Animals ritual, 135–37
flames, 29
floral mandalas, 48–49
free radicals, 122

GABA, 19
gamma waves, 18
Gam Zu L'Tovah, 53–55
gender, 133
generation Z couples, 12
Glymphatic Cleanse ritual, 124–26
Grand Altar of Your Intuition, 126–28
gratitude, 72, 107–8
growth, 58, 74
Guardians of the Night ritual, 48–50

half-sleep, 99–100
head, 88
heartbeat, 107
heart chakra, 72–73, 102
heart coherence, 108–11
heart rate, 16
Heart's Smile ritual, 149–50
Hinduism, 51
homeostasis, 14–15
hormones, 15
house, 38–40
hypnagogia, 99–100
hypothalamus, 19

illness, 69–70
Imperial City ritual, 78–79
Industrial Revolution, 11, 22

In Love With Your House ritual, 38–40
inner alchemy, 18
intangible zone, 34–36
    Cerebral Pathways ritual, 42–44
    Guardians of the Night ritual, 48–50
    In Love With Your House ritual, 38–40
    Let Your Tongue Loose ritual, 40–42
    Liberation of Beings ritual, 46–48
    Nocturnal Feng Shui ritual, 36–38
    Only You Can Do It ritual, 44–46
intention, 8
intimacy, 123–24
intuition, 1–2, 74, 123–24, 135
Ishinfuran, 141–43

Jing, 18
jiva bandha, 41
joy, 73
judgment, fear of, 11–12
Jung, Carl, 35

Keep the Faith Strong ritual, 130–33
Kikuchi, Daisuke, 122
kirtan, 63
Kobayashi, Masaki, 122
kundalini, 159
Kybalion, 132

Lakota prayer, 66
Laniakea ritual, 173–74
learning, 16
letting go, 98
Let Your Tongue Loose ritual, 40–42

Liberation of Beings ritual, 46–48
light, 15, 152–53
Light of the World ritual, 152–53
Lokah Samastha Sukhino, 55–56
lotus flower, 60, 131
love, 107
lucid dreaming, 20–21, 25–27, 91–92
    Clear the Right Nostril ritual, 94–96
    Lucid Meditators ritual, 100–102
    Mnemonic Technique ritual, 93–94
    Nine Round ritual, 96–98
    Palace of Flexibility ritual, 104–6
    Three R's of Lucid Dreaming ritual, 103–4
    Wake up Early ritual, 99–100
Lucid Meditators ritual, 100–102
lymphatic system, 88–89

magic carpet, 140–41
malas, 62–64
male physiology, 11–12
mandalas, 48–49
mantras, 51–52. *See also specific mantras*
marriage, 34
matrimonial bed, 11–12
mattresses, 8–10, 23
Meadows, Robert, 13
meditation, 100–102
medulla oblongata, 19
melatonin, 20, 74, 134–35
Memento Mori ritual, 172–73
memory, 9
memory consolidation, 16
memory storage, 16
menstruation, 72

mental body, 14
mentalism, 132
metabolism, 15, 74, 133
metaconsciousness, 20
metal beds, 10
metal element, 38
midbrain, 19
millennial couples, 12
mindfulness, 58
mirrors, 85
Mnemonic Technique ritual, 93–94
Modeh Ani, 32
mood, 16
moral expectations, 11–12
morphic resonance, 65
morphological field, 65
mudras, 151–52
mula bandha, 77
mysticism, 4

National Sleep Foundation, 12
neck, 88
neidan, 18
new woman, the, 11
night, 33, 48–50
Nine Round ritual, 96–98
Nocturnal Feng Shui ritual, 36–38
Nocturnal Heart ritual, 109–11
Nocturnal Mirror of the Soul, 83–85
Nocturnal Wild Side ritual, 162–64
Noor, 62–64

Om Mani Padme Hum, 59–61
Oneironaut ritual, 25–27
Only You Can Do It ritual, 44–46
Opening Ritual, 2
ovaries, 72
oxytocin, 158
Palace of Flexibility ritual, 104–6
paralysis, 16
partners, 4–5, 22
patience, 94
pelvic floor, 76–77
perineum, 77
personality, 113
personal space, 10
physical body, 14
pillows, 12, 23–24
pineal gland, 19–20, 74, 134–35
pituitary gland, 74
Plato's Cave ritual, 166–69
pleasure. *See* sensuality
pneuma, 18
polarity, 132
pons, 19
Powerful Sleeping Beauty ritual, 117–19
prana, 96
prefrontal cortex, 21

Qi, 18
qigong, 18

Rainbow ritual, 169–71
reasoning, 9
rebirth, 58
refuge, 147–48
REM sleep, 9, 15–17, 100
Repayment ritual, 164–66
reproduction, 74
research, 12–14

rhythm, 132
Richardson, B. W., 10–11
root chakra, 71, 74–75

sacral chakra, 2, 71–72
Sacred Sacrum ritual, 75–77
sacrum, 31
saliva, 4, 81, 120
Sanjiao, 144
Sa Ta Na Ma, 56–59
second chakra, 2, 71–72, 127
Seeking Nocturnal Refuge ritual, 147–48
self-compassion, 94
Self-Embrace ritual, 119–20
self-hypnosis, 109
self-knowledge, 21
Self-Ovation ritual, 144–47
self-reflection, 21
sensuality, 69–70
  ascending chakras, 70–75
  Clitoris ritual, 85–87
  Eroticism Everywhere ritual, 87–90
  Imperial City ritual, 78–79
  Nocturnal Mirror of the Soul, 83–85
  Sacred Sacrum ritual, 75–77
  Sunlight Between Your Legs ritual, 82–83
  Vibrators and Vibrations ritual, 80–91
Sephirot ritual, 159–62
Seven Laws, The, 132–33
seven-year cycles, 70–75
sex, 13
shared beds, 10–11

sheets, 12, 23
Shen, 18
showers, 7–8
sinoatrial node, 118
Sit on the Throne, Queen ritual, 30–32
sleep, stages of, 14–17
Sleep and Depression Laboratory, 13
sleep divorce, 13
sleeping alone
  alternatives, 7–8
  be your own researcher, 12–14
  in defense of, 4–5
  impact on thinking, 19–20
  implementing, 5–6
sleep-wake homeostasis, 14–15
snoring, 12
SoHam, 67–68
solar plexus chakra, 72
solitary space, 4
sound, 149–50
Sovereign of Yin ritual, 137–39
sovereignty, 4, 154–56
Speak Softly to Yourself ritual, 32–33
spine, 105–6
spiritual awakening, 74
stages of sleep, 14
Sunlight Between Your Legs ritual, 82–83
surrender, 3
Surrey Sleep Research Center, 13
symbolism, 35
sympathetic nervous system, 107–8

taboos, 34
testicles, 72
thalamus, 19

theta waves, 18
third eye, 60
third eye chakra, 29, 73–74, 134
three gates, 143–44
Three R's of Lucid Dreaming ritual, 103–4
throat chakra, 73
throne, 30–32
thymus, 72
Tibetan Yogas of Dream and Sleep, The, 82
tongue, 40–42
trachea, 80–81
Trataka ritual, 28–30
Tree of Life, 159–62
true essence, 58

uterine altars, 2
uterus, 2, 127–28

vaginal canal, 80–81
vagus nerve, 81, 150

vessel of information, 1–2
vibration, 132
Vibrators and Vibrations ritual, 80–81
Viparita Karani Mudra, 151–52
Visionary ritual, 112–14
visualization, 28
vocal cords, 80–81

wakefulness, 15
Wake Up Early ritual, 99–100
waking consciousness, 20–21
waterbeds, 10
water element, 38
wealth, 9–10
West, 28
wild side, 162–64
women, power of, 140–41
wood element, 37

Zak, Cynthia, poetry of, 35–36
zikr, 63